MAGNUSON, WARREN GRANT, 1905-
　　HOW MUCH FOR HEALTH? / WARREN G. MAGNUSON AND ELLIOT A.
SEGAL.　WASHINGTON : R. B. LUCE, [1974]
　　XII, 210 P. ;

L.C. CLASSIFICATION: RA410.53.M33
L.C. CARD NUMBER: 747834
-? CLEAR FORMAT
-? SET ELE SA
-? TYPE

SA:
SASU = DRUG TRADE - UNITED STATES.;
SASU = DRUGS - PRICES AND SALE.;
SASU = DRUGS - LAW AND LEGISLATION - UNITED STATES

How Much For Health?

Senator Warren G. Magnuson
and Elliot A. Segal

HOW MUCH
FOR HEALTH?

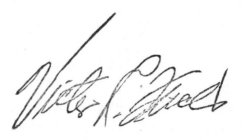

Robert B. Luce, Inc.   Washington–New York

Library of Congress Catalog Card Number 74–7834
ISBN 0–88331–068–6

Contents

Foreword

This book is the product of the mind and heart of a distinguished and compassionate United States Senator who has devoted a major portion of his thirty-eight years in Congress to the promotion of legislation to improve the health of the American people. Senator Warren G. Magnuson understands the essential importance of medical research as a means of providing better health care for the people. No matter what we do or how much we spend to provide better delivery of health care, the *quality* will not improve, and the health of the people will therefore not improve, until we have additional knowledge. That knowledge can come only from research into ways of controlling diseases more effectively, and indeed, preventing them. The cure, control, and prevention of disease are therefore essential means to the advancement of the quality of medical care. Because Senator Magnuson understands this basic concept, he has fought valiantly and indefatigably for the support of medical research.

In 1937, when he first took his seat as a member of the House of Representatives, with his colleague, the late Senator Homer Bone of Washington, he introduced a bill to create a National Cancer Institute. At that time, federal support of medical research was regarded as heretical. Although similar legislation had been proposed as early as 1928, it had always been defeated. The 1937 legislation was passed, and a whole new era of governmental support for medical research against the major fatal diseases of our time was inaugurated.

At the time of passage of the historic cancer legislation, only one in seven victims of cancer was being saved. Today more than one and a half million Americans have survived the ravages of cancer, and this number has been increasing each year. We are now saving one in three victims of cancer and according to the National Cancer Institute and the American Cancer Society, one in two victims could be saved if we applied, to all our people, the knowledge we have acquired from research through the years. This year, the National Cancer Institute is operating on a budget of about $600 million, and the authorized budget for 1975 is $800 million.

In my specialty, cardiovascular disease, establishment of a National Heart Institute in 1948, with Senator Magnuson as one of the chief sponsors of the legislation, opened a vigorous offensive against a disease which claims a million American lives each year. On many occasions when I have had the privilege of testifying before the Senate Appropriations Committee on which Senator Magnuson serves, I have pointed out that the remarkable progress we have made against cardiovascular disease almost exactly parallels the growth of the National Heart Institute — a rate of progress which during this past quarter century has exceeded that made in all previous recorded history.

For example, a decade ago the incidence of in-hospital deaths from heart attacks was about thirty percent. In the best heart centers today, this figure has dropped to as low as six percent. Surgical procedures are now available for the correction of almost all congenital heart defects, even in early infancy. Open heart surgery and other procedures have restored thousands upon thousands of Americans, formerly doomed to death, to lives of productivity and happiness. Aneurysms of the aorta, valvular disease, and various forms of occlusive disease of the arteries, including those of the coronaries, which cause more deaths than all others combined, are now being better managed by surgical procedures that were not available ten years ago. Before the development of these new operations through medical research, these patients were doomed to certain death.

We still have a long way to go, however. In 1972, the National Health and Lung Act required that the administration develop a five-year plan for the eventual conquest of a disease which kills two Americans every minute. That plan, released last year, estimated that heart and lung diseases alone cost the nation $40 billion a year. It concluded that a national gain of about eleven years in life expectancy would occur if all cardiac and vascular diseases could be eliminated or ameliorated.

As the president of one of the largest medical schools in the country, I am deeply concerned about the proposal to eliminate all research training programs. For more than two decades Congress has recognized, and given support to, the need to train the young research scientists and clinicians who will produce the new knowledge we need to move ahead. As chairman of the Senate Appropriations Subcommittee on Labor-HEW, Senator Magnuson was a key figure in restoring these funds and in getting the Congress this year to pass legislation authorizing specific monies for research training and fellowships over the next three years.

In addition to being compassionate, Senator Magnuson is persevering. He uses every ethical means to further the health programs in which he deeply believes. For example, in 1973 Labor-HEW bills were twice vetoed on the grounds that the proposed funding for medical research was excessive, and $1.1 billion in funds appropriated for health were impounded. The senior Senator from Washington did not despair. Over a period of many months, he and his staff searched for documentation that these funds had been requested by the various directors of the National Institutes of Health as vital to any forward movement in medical research. When the data had been accumulated, he and his distinguished colleague, Senator Mike Mansfield, the Majority Leader of the Senate, held a series of conferences which ultimately led to restoration of the funds.

Space does not permit a listing of his many other achievements in the health field. In the decade during which he served as chairman of the Appropriations Subcommittee which dealt with the Veterans Administration, almost single-handedly he raised the appropriation for medical research in the Veterans Administration from less than $4 million to more than $50 million. More recently he was the chief sponsor of the National Health Service Corps, a measure designed to bring physicians and other paramedical professionals into the underserved city and rural low-income areas of this country.

His work in the field of national health insurance is less known to the American people. For more than three decades he has been a supporter of the principle that every American must have the financial means to purchase high quality health services. In the early years of this crusade, his and many other voices were drowned out by the accusation that he was advocating "Socialized Medicine". In 1974 it seems that the time has finally come for acceptance of the concept of national health insurance. There is little doubt that this goal will finally be reached.

In October 1973, I had the honor of speaking at a dinner in Seattle at which Senator Magnuson received the coveted Albert Lasker Public Service Award for Leadership in Health. This award, frequently referred to as the "American Nobel Prize in Medicine", has been given to only four legislators in the twenty-seven years of its existence. I closed my remarks with this admonition of Benjamin Disraeli, spoken almost one hundred years ago:

The health of the people is really the foundation upon which all their happiness and all their powers as a State depend.

Senator Magnuson has followed to a passionate degree the admonition of Mr. Disraeli. This book is an illustration of what we must do to bring the bounty of good health within the reach of every American whatever be his race, creed, or economic status.

Michael E. DeBakey, M.D.
President, Baylor College of Medicine
Houston, Texas

Introduction

For the sick and diseased, the restoration of health is the overriding concern of their lives. For the healthy, the threat of illness and disease, while less immediate, remains a "brooding omnipresence." While good health and the absence of disease is always a central *private* concern, it is only in the last few decades that it has emerged as a central *public* concern. Yet two hundred years ago we pledged our society to safeguarding "life, liberty and the pursuit of happiness." Is there any human condition which more directly and poignantly denies to us those inalienable rights than dread disease and inadequate health care?

A government which does not direct its energies to the eradication of disease or injury and does not provide its citizens with basic health care is as derelict as that government was from which we declared our independence almost 200 years ago. As a United States Senator, I have tried to influence government actions to improve the health of every man, woman, and child in this country. I am proud that health research in the United States is second to none. And I recognize that many of the world's most sophisticated clinics and hospitals are in American cities. But I have been, and continue to be, concerned about current government directions toward health care and spending priorities which allocate more than a third of the federal budget for the machinery of war and death rather than the assurance of health for all of our citizens.

Our purpose in writing this book is to discuss with the American people the present state of health care in this country, outline certain goals which we think must be attained, and point to specific government actions, some of which are facilitating the attainment of those goals, and others of which are retarding their attainment. It is my hope that the words on the pages which follow will stimulate the people of this country to demand of their government those actions necessary to secure for each individual the right to reasonable health care. It is also my hope that, through the examples of specific governmental activities which are discussed, those interested in working for the attainment of reasonable health care for all citizens will gain some perspective and insight into how they can work through the political process to attain that objective.

A consistent theme throughout this book is how government policy affects the pocketbooks of the health care consumer and how there is a need for the health care consumer to assert himself in government policy-making and in management of the health care system.

My own involvement in the consumer movement convinces me that, when the American citizen as consumer of goods and services makes his voice heard, then constructive governmental and market responses result.

Because health care has been historically wrapped in a medical mystique, it is seldom looked upon as a product to be purchased. Nevertheless, there is probably no more valuable product that we can buy and sell in our daily lives. Consumer knowledge and consumer demands for changes can be a potent force for attaining appropriate health care in the United States. It is for that reason that we have consistently stressed the consumer perspective in this book.

In the hope of facilitating the purposes of this book, we have divided it into two basic parts. The first part of the book assesses the current state of health, examines health care priorities, and criticizes present government policies. Three case studies are used to illustrate the centrality that health research plays in a health care system, and the role which government can play in preventing accidental injury and disease. Thus, Chapter 4 discusses the war on cancer, now three years old, and the problems involved since its implementation. Chapter 6 discusses the establishment of a Consumer Product Safety Commission and its injury prevention mission, and Chapter 5 discusses new initiatives in the environmental health area (safe drinking water, toxic substances control, and no-fault insurance) which can have important salutary effects upon the nation's health care problems.

In the second part of the book, we present and discuss what we believe are the essential ingredients of a comprehensive and coordinated health care system. Chapters 7 through 12 lay out the six ingredients which we believe are necessary for a total health care system. Particular attention is paid to the needs which have already been met in each of the program areas, and the directions that must be pressed over the next decade. In these chapters we attempt to indicate ways in which the needed integration of the essential elements can be accomplished in order to produce a coordinated policy and action plan for health care delivery in the United States.

In the second part of the book, there is a necessary expansion of the material contained in the first part of the book. For example, the way to dramatically improve government action to prevent injury to the health of our citizens is discussed in Chapters 5 and 6 and again in Chapter 12. While these chapters illustrate similar points, we have used different examples to illustrate to the reader the wide variety of governmental activities which can have a positive impact upon health care in the United States, The examples of lead paint, fire prevention and control, and food safety included in Chapter 12 should indicate how much more we have to accomplish in the entire area of health consumer protection over the next decade.

There are many people who have contributed substantially to the making of this book. I am grateful to the hundreds of witnesses who have come before the Senate to testify and who have presented important suggestions that help shape legislation. I am also grateful to the thousands of average citizens who take the trouble to write me and let me

xi

know their ideas and thoughts on federal programs. At this particular time, when confidence in government is being tested, it is heartening to see such concern for working with the processes of government.

I am deeply grateful for the dedicated staff assistance I have received in this effort. This includes my personal staff as well as individuals serving with the Commerce Committee and Health Appropriations Subcommittee. The Library of Congress and the National Library of Medicine have also been quite helpful. I am particularly indebted to William Prochnau and Lynn Sutcliffe for their critical comments and editing of the manuscript. I am, as always, grateful to my wife Jermaine, who is a constant source of inspiration and assistance to me.

Warren G. Magnuson
United States Senator

1   The Present

Health care in the United States needs to be improved. The American people must be guaranteed the best care available, when needed and without being limited by cost. It is useful to examine health issues in six areas of national concern. These are research, costs, organization, quality, manpower and facilities, and prevention of environmental health hazards.

Research

Medical research belongs at the top of the list of national concerns. Research holds the key that will someday unlock the mysteries of disease, and the hope that such illnesses as cancer and heart disease can ultimately be cured as a result. We are just now beginning to see the fruits of some of the early efforts.

A disease area such as "crib death" requires research at the earliest and most basic levels. The following letters have been addressed to members of Congress by parents of victims of "crib death", more technically known as the Sudden Infant Death Syndrome (SIDS).

New York

Dear Sirs: I have just finished reading a story in a magazine about "crib death." I can't begin to tell you how much I appreciated it. On April 16, 1969 we lost our seven week old baby. Coroner's Report: Crib Death. I had heard little about these deaths, still we searched magazines, newspapers for anything we could find on the subject, anything to enlighten us to the facts about these deaths. I kept asking myself, did I do anything wrong? Did I overfeed him, should I have laid him on his back instead of his stomach, will this happen again? All kinds of endless, torturing questions.

. . .You'd be surprised how ignorant the general public is about this, people would ask us what did your baby die from and when we would say SIDS they'd look at us like we were crazy. . . . The Coroner showed us a clipping that he carried in his wallet about these deaths, he told us that he had seen marriages break up because one mate would blame the other, why? because most people don't know or have never read about crib death.

Please tell us how we can help others to understand.

Missouri

Dear sirs: I need your help. My 2 month daughter has died and I love her very much. It was our first child. She was born on January 31, 1971 — she died April 1, 1971.

My baby — I carried her for nine months. She weighed 8 pounds, 2½ ounces she never lost any weight she gained. When she died she weighed 14 pounds and was very happy. She ate good, slept good.

Our family got the flu. I was wondering if my baby could of gotten the flu without anyone knowing about it. The only thing that happened was that I did not realize till she died that for three days before she died she slept 2 days and I had to wake her up to feed her. Then the next day she was alright. That night I gave her supper then I put her to bed. She seemed restless but everybody told me that lots of babies do cry all night and are all right. She had just been for a check up and she was alright. Well, I picked her up and rocked her to sleep. She was breathing okay. She didn't act like she had a cold or anything. The next morning she was dead.

Now I am a nervous wreck. I don't care if I live or not. The man that checks dead people said there was no sense in doing anything to her because they won't find anything. I am heartbroken.

What I want to know is do you have any idea what could have been wrong with her? They told me it might be "crib death" — what is that — I don't believe that my baby or any baby could die from nothing.

We want to have more children but I am scared to become pregnant because I am afraid it will happen again. I just can't take it anymore. I am on nerve pills. I keep hearing her crying. I don't feel like seeing my friends because when I do I don't know what to say to them. I need your help. I am going to end up in a mental hospital if I don't get some help from someone soon. I am so lonely.

These letters demonstrate the pain, anguish, and despair that accompany this completely unexpected tragedy. In order to make progress against the mysterious "crib death", we need to commit money for research. There is also a need for better understanding of the needs of the bereaved parents. At present, so little is known about this disease that parents have been locked up in jail, suspected of killing their own babies. It is government's responsibility to support the necessary research. The causes of the disease are unknown and answers appear to be far off.

A total health program is needed, of which health research must be an essential ingredient. There are many more areas that require research, including multiple sclerosis, cerebral palsy, diabetes, and sickle cell anemia, among others. Understanding of such diseases does not come easily — the task of underwriting the basic research must be taken on by the federal government. For example, researchers think that "crib death" may be caused by a virus; scientists need the money to explore this possibility. We would never have been able to identify the virus that causes polio without a good program of basic research.

Costs

Medical costs continue to skyrocket. The cost of care to the average health consumer is moving out of the range of his or her ability to pay. Even worse are situations where cost becomes the only factor that determines who gets care and who does not. The story of Jody Dietrich is an example.

Henry Dietrich earns a modest $125 a week at his job exercising horses at a race track not far from his Broward County home in Davie, Florida. When doctors told him that his oldest son Jody, 6, was suffering from a serious heart defect that would require treatment costing $2,500, Dietrich was hard pressed to come up with the money. What's more, he apparently misunderstood hospital administrators when they told him that they would appreciate a deposit before admitting his son. They were not demanding any money in advance, they said later. But no matter, Dietrich told friends about his plight, and a women's service sorority promptly set up the Jody Dietrich Heart Surgery Fund.

The fund languished, however, until last week, when a thin blonde woman in her early 20's walked into Davie's Sterling National Bank, mumbled something to a secretary, and left a package addressed to Robert Ruckman, the bank's president and the chief collector for the fund. In the package were $2,000 in twenty, fifty and one hundred dollar bills and a letter explaining the gift: "WHAT THE HELL IS HAPPENING IN THIS COUNTRY WHEN A SIX-YEAR-OLD CHILD NEEDS LIFE-SAVING SURGERY AND IS DENIED TREATMENT BECAUSE SOME HOSPITAL DEMANDS A DOWN PAYMENT ON THE INHERENT RIGHT HE WAS BORN WITH TO HEALTH AND HAPPINESS? We are enclosing $2,000, which we hope will give Jody Dietrich at least a small shot at life, and we soundly condemn people in the system who made this action on our part necessary, although we do it gladly." (TIME Magazine — Dec. 10, 1973)

4

Few stories such as Jody Dietrich's appear in national magazines, but similar dramas occur every day. In order to turn health care into a right for American citizens and not a privilege for the few, the cost factor must be eliminated.

The problem of high costs could be alleviated by good health insurance coverage, but insurance companies may use legal maneuvers and loopholes to get around payments. The following case was presented in evidence during the 1972 hearings before the Senate Judiciary Subcommittee on Anti-Trust and Monopoly.

A 50-year-old female confined to a hospital from February 18, 1972 to March 17, 1972 had had insurance with a company since October 1970. In answer to the company's first inquiry to the physician as to the nature of the illness, the physician reported on April 17, 1972 that the patient was admitted for obesity and congestive heart failure, and that the congestive heart failure was a new diagnosis, not pre-existing. The company wrote to the doctor again and requested his opinion on how many days of the patient's confinement could be attributed to the treatment of obesity. The doctor replied on May 15, 1972 that there was no way to separate the conditions, i.e. congestive heart failure and obesity.

The company then rejected the claim on the grounds of a pre-existing condition; namely, that the lady was obese prior to the time that she purchased the policy.

It is estimated that the month's stay in the hospital brought this woman a bill for over $5,000. Seventeen months of paying insurance premiums had done her no good. Better and more truthful public information would help consumers be better protected against $5,000 bills for congestive heart failure.

Eliminating the loopholes and co-insurances and deductibles is even more important. There is no better example than that very ordinary common need for hospitalization, the happy event of a child being born. But these days the high cost of such an event subtracts significantly from the joy.

The Washington Star in 1970 had a series on the high costs of health. Judith Randal wrote the following:

Last month, Mary S., a typical suburban wife and mother, brought her second child, a boy, home from a Washington hospital. The charges for her four-day stay in a semi-private room and the uncomplicated delivery and circumcision of the baby came to $360.

Two years earlier, Mrs. S. had made an almost identical trip to the hospital for the delivery of her first-born, also a boy. When she checked out that time, the bill was $273. What had happened between late 1967 and late 1969 to increase the cost of a routine obstetrical case by more than 31%, while the cost of living in the Washington area was increasing by only 11%?

If Mrs. S. makes a similar trip to the hospital in 1974, the cost shock will be even greater. An identical routine obstetrical case at the same hospital for the delivery of another boy could cost over $500.

It is because of costs like these that Congress has been actively debating the establishment of a national health insurance program. Rapidly rising costs led Congress in 1965 to establish Medicare, a program that would pay for hospitalization of our elderly citizens. But with health care expenses escalating so quickly, government must act to assure that all other needy portions of our population receive quality health care regardless of price.

Organization

The delivery of health care in this country is also a problem. Sometimes care is denied to a person who does not fit into a certain income eligibility category. One of the most striking examples was the story behind the blaring headline, "Couple To Get Divorce To Gain Medicaid Help". Judy McKnight, writing for the *St. Petersburg Evening Independent* in January 1973, gave the following description of the plight of Howard and Ruth Thomas:

A St. Petersburg man is divorcing his wife in a last ditch effort to get her the state aid she needs to stay alive.

The 45-year-old woman, a multiple sclerosis victim confined to the Beverly Manor Convalescent Center, recently lost her Medicaid benefits because of financial ineligibility.

Her husband, a steelworker in Tampa, takes home approximately $550 a month. The state's maximum for eligibility is $427 and is based on what it would cost to give nursing care in the home: $119 for basic personal hospital needs, $62 for shelter and $246 for nursing care.

The man in tears yesterday told of his intensive search for help and funding. He has made several trips to Tallahassee only to be referred to local agencies that say they cannot help him.

. . ."I love my wife, and it won't make any difference to me that we are divorced. But, if that's the only way she can get care, then I'll have to accept it."

. . ."It's a sad day when a person has to get a divorce in order to receive care." said Boyd Hendrickson, administrator of the nursing home.

But no one, other than the Legal Aid attorney the man was sent to, could come up with a solution.

Because the woman has no income herself, a divorce would mean that she probably would become financially eligible for state aid. The Division of Family Services does not guarantee this but the husband already has asked a social worker to begin a new application, this time for his wife as a single individual.

"We're all upset about this," said the attorney's secretary, "but we couldn't see any other way to help this man. I hope you can do something."

. . ."Why is it that the average man gets hurt?" asked the husband. "If I were real poor or real rich, I could take care of my wife. I work hard for a living and this is what happens. I just don't understand."

The couple has two small children, aged 5 and 11, who are staying with married sisters. Until recently, the father was paying $30 a week for their care. He has discontinued those payments because he doesn't have the money.

"I'm trying to pay off the nursing home bills, but I just can't do it alone."

His balance is $2,892.14. On Feb. 1, however, he will receive another bill and the average monthly cost to care for his wife is about $800 to $1,000 a month.

A trust fund was established at the St. Petersburg Commercial Bank, 2100 34th St. S, with Mrs. Margaret Ryden. However, the donations have not been for more than $400.

"There is no other answer," the man said. "I'm going to get the divorce in order to help my wife, but I want to thank all of those who have thought and helped us during this unbelievable period."

Addendum: Wife Divorced to Qualify for Aid Dies
(St. Petersburg, Fla., Dec. 14, 1973 (AP)

Ruth Thomas, divorced by her husband 10 months ago so she could qualify for state medical aid, has died of multiple sclerosis.

Mrs. Thomas' seven-year battle with the debilitating disease ended Wednesday night at Welkind Neurological Center in Chester, N.J.

"She suffered so long I guess it's for the best," said steelworker Howard Thomas. "She's better off now."

Something is wrong with our health care system when a couple, obviously in love, has to obtain a divorce in order to allow the wife to receive medical help.

While, as the Thomas family situation indicates, health care can be withheld because of arbitrary categorical distinctions, it may also be denied because the person does not have the available cash. This situation must be changed.

The federal government must take a more active role in the organization and delivery of health services. The American public needs to know that its government will assure that adequate care will be available to people when they need it.

Standards

It is not enough just to make sure that care is available. There need to be standards to protect the consumer and insure the quality of service that is dispensed. In a November 1972 *Washington Post* series, Ronald Kessler described how the chief physicians at a major Washington, D.C. hospital were afraid of their own product (surgical operations) because of the quality of their anesthesiologists.

"I was very scared when my daughter came up for routine surgery (at the Washington Hospital Center) last spring" confides Dr. Richard C. Reba, chief of the center's nuclear medicine department, which diagnoses illnesses by tracing the path of radioactive substances introduced into the blood stream.

The latest anesthesia accidents in the center's operating rooms are commonly the subject of discussion when doctors at the hospital gather for lunch, according to Dr. Reba. He further says that he would not allow his daughter to enter the center for surgery until the surgeon assured him that he only uses a certain two of the hospital's anesthesiologists.

Dr. Ernest A. Gould, former chief of the medical staff and chief of surgery until 1970, says he would only allow four of the more than twenty anesthesiologists at the center to give him anesthesia if he had to undergo an operation.

Even if it were an emergency, he wouldn't allow two of the anesthesiologists (one of whom has recently left the hospital) to go near him, nor would he allow them in an operating room with him while he was performing surgery.

Samuel Scrivener, Jr., president of the Hospital Center, says the problem is that many anesthesiologists are trained in foreign countries and cannot speak English well. Instant communication between anesthesiologist and surgeon is essential throughout an operation, says Dr. Gould. Referring to the language problem, Dr. Gould adds: "If the answer requires a 'yes' or 'no', they're o.k. But if it involves an explanation, they need help."

9

This example of quality focuses on the competence of the practitioners. Congressman Tim Lee Carter, a physician himself and a member of the House of Representatives Health Subcommittee, declared in August 1973 that he had known many fine foreign doctors, "but make no mistake about it, I prefer the American brand."

A 1972 study commissioned by the Department of Health, Education, and Welfare (HEW) concluded that "a growing body of evidence indicates that as a total group, and for whatever reasons, foreign medical graduates do less well on standard tests than their American counterparts." The American Medical Association (AMA) gathered statistics in 1972 showing that students from foreign medical schools failed licensing tests 36.2 percent of the time while American students had an 11.3 percent rate. There may be little opportunity to choose a competent, trained physician. It is rare to know even the name of the anesthesiologist in the surgical room during one's own operation, yet one's life is in his or her hands. Someone must ensure the availability of qualified doctors.

The need for better trained doctors is only one example of what is required to protect the consumer and to guarantee high quality. Unnecessary procedures and obsolete, inadequate facilities and equipment are other factors.

Manpower

There are several hundred communities in this country that need a physician but do not have one. Many people have come to us in Congress to describe the dire consequences of having no immediate medical care available. The unfortunate story of Wolcott, Indiana, as told by CBS reporter Daniel Schorr in 1970, is a good example:

Wolcott, Indiana: Is There a Doctor in the Town?
Bob Foster, the local funeral director, is an important man in life as well as death. His hearse has done double duty as an ambulance to take the stricken to the doctor, sometimes as far as thirty miles away. Wolcott, a

comfortable town of 8,000, living off the land, can easily afford a doctor, but like 5,000 small communities in the hustings, it has trouble getting one. Today, with 8,000 doctors a year coming out of medical school, few choose to treat patients, and most of these few prefer to live in the cities or in the suburbs. So, for two years, Wolcott had no doctor.

Correspondent George Herman heard the consequences of this in conversations in Nordyke's Drug Store, the chief local center for health care.

A woman said, "We had a five-year-old boy that got sick in the middle of the night. And then, I think, that's when you really notice most that you can't get any help. I couldn't get a doctor to come to the house, so we just had to take him to the hospital in Lafayette."

A man said, "When I don't feel well, I come to Doc Nordyke, and I say, 'Doc, you gotta fix me up.' and he gives me something."

Pharmacist Bob Nordyke said, "They used to go to the doctor with their ailments. Now they come in and say, 'What do you have for the twenty-four hour flu?' and that sort of thing. I think that my major job is to tell them that I've got something for them that will help, or say, 'Your problem is a little too serious, and you'd better get in touch with the doctor.' "

For emergencies there is Bob Foster. Then it's a thirty-mile ride in the hearse-ambulance to the hospital in Lafayette.

Some residents told their problems in the local tavern.

"I had a man working for me, and he had a coronary heart attack at seven o'clock in the morning. It was winter and pitch dark. And before anything could be done for him, he was dead. I feel that if there had been a doctor available, that man would have been alive today. He was thirty-nine years old. . . ."

"I went to a doctor in Rensselaer. The man's got more than he can take care of. You go to Remington,

11

and they turn you down. You just can't get any help. In all those places you're lucky if you can get in to see the doctor."

The citizens of Wolcott appealed to the Indiana State medical school, largest in the country. They wrote to every intern in every hospital in the state. They advertised in newspapers as far away as Chicago. They flew banners over football games reading, "Wolcott Needs a Doctor!". And they kept an office vacant, hoping to find a young physician to fill it.

On one occasion, the dean of the state medical school and a medical student came to answer anxious questions at a town meeting. As to the chance of getting a doctor, the student told them bluntly:

"I think its kind of poor. I think its not just poor for this town, but for many small towns across the nation that are trying to get physicians. It isn't money, and it is only partially what the community has to offer. The doctor is really no different from any other professional. My colleagues want better hours."

Having enough doctors now and in the future is not our only manpower problem. We are also heading for a major nursing shorage.

In March 1973, the director of nursing at the Department of Health, Education and Welfare (HEW) sent a position paper to the director of the Bureau of Health Manpower Education. It contained a warning that the proposed Nixon Administration budget cuts would:

1. Put an "immediate brake" on the trend toward increasing enrollments in nursing schools and thereby intensify the nursing shortage.
2. Speed up the closing of some education programs and force the closing of others.
3. Dangerously reduce the number of registered nurses being prepared for teaching and administrative roles.
4. Result in an immediate termination of all on-going nursing research and a complete halt in all new nursing

research — ending a 19-year-old program which has made major contributions to the saving of lives in such areas as coronary disease, tuberculosis, brain disease and kidney disease.

5. Reduce the efforts to bring minorities and disadvantaged people into nursing and have a crippling effect on the efforts to alleviate the nursing shortages in under-served areas.

These facts were uncovered by the General Accounting Office (GAO) and the Library of Congress when they examined the impact of the Nixon Administration 1974 budget cutbacks. This examination was done at the request of Senator Mike Mansfield and myself.

These examples raise the fundamental question of the proper role of the federal government in the health manpower picture. When nursing and applied health programs were passed in 1971 we were told to expect a national shortage of at least 150,000 nurses by 1980. Cutting back now could only make that prediction inevitable. On learning of these cutbacks, Senator Mansfield and I indicated that it would be foolish to play such games with the health of the American people.

President Nixon openly contradicts himself on the question of the nation's health manpower needs. In 1971 President Nixon stated that "expanded manpower programs are an integral part of the national health strategy. One of the cardinal principles on which this strategy was built was that of balancing the supply of medical care with the growing demand for services. Our failure to achieve this balance can only result in lower quality medical care at increasingly inflated prices." Since making that statement, the President proposed a 43 percent cutback in funds to finance federal health manpower programs.

If thousands of communities such as Wolcott, Indiana cannot get a doctor to practice locally, then this country has a health manpower shortage — no matter what else one chooses to call it. Health care as a right must be extended to the residents of towns without doctors. The federal government has no alternative but to take steps to bring about a solution to this manpower problem.

Environment

Environmental factors play an important role in promoting optimum health. To improve health care we must eliminate, prevent or minimize environmental hazards which are harmful to our health. Without proper respect and control over the adverse effects of various kinds of pollution, for instance, they may expose the public to unnecessary physical and physiological dangers. A team of investigators at the Medical College of Wisconsin led by Dr. Richard D. Stewart released a report in December 1973 concluding that many Americans are regularly exposed to carbon monoxide. Carbon monoxide is, of course, a colorless, odorless, tasteless, invisible gas which is being linked more and more to heart disease. We are all too familiar with accidental deaths that result from carbon monoxide produced by fires or faulty gas refrigerators and heaters.

The study indicated that while tobacco smoking is the single most important factor leading to raised levels of carbon monoxide, other environmental factors are also important. These include occupational hazards, geography and automobile exhausts.

The researchers stated that:

The most relevant finding to come out of this 30-month study was the astounding observation that 45 percent of all the nonsmoking blood donors tested had carbon monoxide saturations greater than 1.5 percent. The Clean Air Act's quality standards of 1971 set 1.5 percent saturation as the highest safe level for active nonsmokers.

The investigators added:

None of the large urban communities had carbon monoxide concentrations low enough to comply with the

Environmental Protection Agency's ambient air quality standards for carbon monoxide.

Further, the investigators said, "urban dwellers had consistently higher carbon monoxide saturations (blood levels) than did their counterparts from adjacent rural areas". Dr. Richard D. Stewart and his 11 co-investigators said they considered their study to be the largest study evaluating carbon monoxides as an air pollutant. They went on:

> Persons sampled in urban areas with high automobile density consistently had carbon monoxide saturations greater than those measured in persons sampled in areas of low automobile density. This was dramatically evident in the comparison of individuals working on Governor's Island, where the average carbon monoxide saturation was .8 percent, half that of persons donating blood in adjacent New York City areas.

The heart and brain are the organs most vulnerable to the insidious effect of environmental carbon monoxide, which is one of the most lethal poisons known.

Another important environmental hazard is lead poisoning. An HEW Report on Lead Poisoning in Children had the following to say:

> Lead poisoning in children, resulting mostly from ingestion of chips of lead-containing paint from walls and woodwork in old, dilapidated housing, remains a unique public health problem. Its etiology, pathogenesis, patho-physiology, and epidemiology are known. Practical methods are available for screening, diagnosis, prevention, and treatment, Yet each year lead poisoning continues to cause the deaths of many children and mental retardation or other neurological handicaps in many other children.

> Health workers should be reminded, and the public informed, that lead poisoning is preventable. As is true with many other diseases, total prevention may be difficult to achieve, but significant reduction in the number

15

and severity of lead poisoning cases can be expected from a well-planned program.

The late Congressman William F. Ryan, a leading advocate for federal action in this subject, testified on March 9, 1972 before the Senate Subcommittee on Health:

Sometimes it is called the silent epidemic; sometimes it is referred to as ghetto malaria. But no matter what it is called, the tragic fact remains that childhood lead poisoning continues needlessly to plague the children of America. Each year thousands of young children are afflicted by this dread disease. The exact number of youngsters poisoned is unknown, for there are still far too few programs to screen children for lead poisoning. The Department of Health, Education, and Welfare has estimated that each year some 400,000 children are subject to lead-based paint poisoning.

As a result, some 16,000 youngsters require treatment. An additional 3,200 suffer moderate to severe brain damage. And 800 are so severely afflicted that they require institutionalization for the remainder of their lives.

And for another 200 children there is no future at all — not even the vegetable-like existance of permanent institutionalization — for they will die as a result of this crippler of young children. Two hundred children a year.

Health care and consumer health protection must go well beyond ensuring that citizens get medical care when they need it. Personal medical services should be considered as a major ingredient of health that is guaranteed to the public. But of equal concern to consumers is the need to have clean air and clean water and to have their health, safety, and welfare protected against environmental hazards.

It is important for government to ensure and for citizens to know the advantages of programs such as no-fault automobile insurance. Because of the annual carnage on our turnpikes and roads, and because of an antiquated liability system of covering individuals who are unfortunate enough to

16

be hurt in accidents, a no-fault insurance program could protect the public health as much as discovering a new vaccine against a dread disease. Health care and rehabilitation treatments could be immediate because payment could be assured.

A food inspection program, a safe drinking water program, and a poison materials or toxic substances program are all measures that should be required to protect the health of our citizens. Since many of these problems have now gone far beyond local and state boundaries and resources, the federal government must at least set up standards to protect the consumer.

This is particularly true for consumer products which are manufactured in one given state and then shipped all over the country. The public has often assumed that toys that are sold in stores must be safe. This is not necessarily true. The public has often assumed that clothes for children that make it to the market are safe to wear and will not cause children to become "human torches". This, too, has not necessarily been true. Many of these problems need to be brought to the attention of the public, and this must be followed by the public letting their elected officials know their concern and desire for legislative action.

It is hoped that this book will alert consumers to many of the flaws in our system of providing the best health care we know to the public, and that consumers will use this information in moving toward constructive action.

These six areas of the health care system should illustrate that health care in this country is at a crossroads. People have always discussed the problem from the standpoint that improvements need to be made in the delivery of health care. Others have even gone so far as to call the current situation a crisis. But in the last few years it has taken on an added dimension: the Nixon Administration has made a major effort to cut back rather than increase federal activity in health and medical areas.

Ironically, the current debate has been almost a silent one. It has not taken place within the halls of Congress or within medical schools or even medical societies. In fact, the pullback from health as a right by the Nixon Administration seems to be a decision made without involving, and in some cases against the advice of, health experts. The decision seems to be an attempt to pinch pennies with no consideration for the programs involved, and more importantly, with no consideration for the hardships this will cause the health care consumer.

Never before has there been a national administration that has made a systematic attempt to curtail progress both in research and in health care delivery. Now Congress and the public have to come to grips with a whole new road map to ensure that medical care be made available to everyone. It seems pure folly to cut back in areas in which we have become world-renowned, such as medical research through the National Institutes of Health (NIH), which is the research section of HEW. Congress and the public have taken justifiable pride in NIH, which, both at its Bethesda, Maryland complex and in supported research throughout the country, has produced some of the most important medical breakthroughs in recent medical history. These breakthroughs have been in applied research leading to immediate help to the citizens of the world, as well as in basic research. NIH has supported several scientists who have won Nobel Prizes for their research achievements. It is foolish to penny-pinch and attempt a cutback (as the Nixon Administration has) in eight of the ten research institutes at NIH. The goal of such centers of research is to resolve the many questions that must be answered so that more lives can be saved and human suffering and hardships can be lessened. The benefits of research breakthroughs are enormous when compared to the small amount of money invested. The research breakthroughs in polio are a good example.

A measure of our commitment to health can be found in the health budget. Recently the federal budget has become more widely recognized as a reflection of national policy. The Urban Coalition in 1971 published a counterbudget which attempted to focus national debate on a shifting of priorities,

18

particularly from defense spending to domestic areas.

The Brookings Institution has also become involved in a series of studies on the federal budget as an expression of national policy. Their most recent analysis underlines how the current administration is attempting to redirect fundamental changes in national policy by making substantive cuts in domestic programs. Cutbacks in health appear to be a part of this fundamental shift.

Movement by the Nixon Administration away from health programs led Senator Mike Mansfield, Senate Majority Leader, and me to call in the General Accounting Office (GAO) and the Library of Congress to study the consequences of these cutbacks. I felt compelled to take this step after four vetoes of HEW budget bills which I had authored. All of my proposals had attempted to give high priority to areas such as medical research. The investigation by GAO and the Library of Congress revealed that many health programs were being plagued by executive impoundment of funds and many other penny-wise but pound-foolish devices.

We must now ask what is the appropriate role that government should play in guaranteeing health care to its citizens. People have always been victims of illness and disease, but there has not usually been the feeling that the government was at fault, or that it was the responsibility of elected officials to alter the situation.

This is changing. The six program areas described above are now becoming areas of national concern. Although health has been of growing concern to elected officials, there has not yet been enough urging by constituents to give it the priority that it deserves. Citizens are only now beginning to express their feeling that health care is a *right* and not a privilege.

It is this kind of demand that will have to be placed on lawmakers by the public before a truly comprehensive health care system will become a reality. It is not enough to pass a few more health bills. This kind of ad hoc response to specific needs (although they cover very important problem areas such as emergency services, or regional medical programs) is only a partial solution.

19

The GAO findings indicate that White House budget officials have even made controversial changes against the advice of HEW's own experts. The HEW scientists and professionals warned that the proposed budget would have a serious impact on the national health care effort.

Congress has begun to take steps at anti-impoundment but a willful and spiteful administration can continue to apply dilatory tactics through unnecessary bureaucratic and administrative requirements. These tactics may force Congress to establish a national statement or policy that transcends the annual budget — but such a policy must have a strong public mandate behind it.

President Kennedy's statement of a national policy and goal in the space effort — the attempt to put a man on the moon by 1970 — certainly inspired great success and helped to gather tremendous support for the space program. A number of national domestic legislative policy statements have been made, but their stated goals have not been met and support has been inconsistent at best. It may be helpful to look at the difference between the space program and other such efforts in order to ferret out the reasons for its success.

The major difference is that the space program captured the imagination and support of the public. This led the public to demand that the resources be voted by Congress to land a man on the moon. There was no question that people expected and wanted government to meet the target within a decade. The "War on Cancer" has not yet received similar public support.

A major "moon shot" effort in cancer or, hopefully, in the entire health area will require unwaning commitment of the public and their elected officials. The public must be sufficiently aware of the need for a broad governmental health program, and in effect be willing to "vote" for its implementation. Just as there is no doubt that the American people accept the fact that public education is a right for every citizen, we need to establish health care as a right and to make it available to all citizens who need it. One of the purposes and hopes of this book is to help that cause along.

The federal government has an immense stake in the health of its citizens. Federal spending for all aspects of health in budget year 1974 exceeded $30 billion, nearly a third of the entire country's expenditure of $94 billion on health. This total amount of $94 billion means an average of $440 was spent on the health of every man, woman, and child in that year. Or, to look at the same figures differently, a family of four had health costs amounting to $1,760, including about $600 that the federal government paid. Yet five years ago, the total bill for that same family would have been $1,200. Uncle Sam's bill would have been $400. Clearly, both the family and government have a stake in keeping health costs down.

But every sign points toward higher health bills for you and Uncle Sam. Projections compiled by the Social Security Administration in 1970 show that the nation will be spending between $156 billion and $189 billion by 1980 if the present rate of increase continues. If that prediction is at all accurate (and recent health cost increases indicate the projections are on target — even with the Cost of Living Council's economic controls) then the average cost for health in 1980 for every man, woman, and child will be in the range of $700 to $800. That means that a family of four without any unusual problems or expenses will be spending over $3,000 a year for health *on the average.*

The cost for any one consumer will of course vary, depending on factors beyond the control of himself or his family. While most families will not have to spend $1,760 per year, others will suffer a serious accident or illness and incur expenses far above the average. Many of these families will lose their life savings and face total ruin, financial and otherwise. You will recall, for example, the family described in Chapter 1, who spent their entire life savings and still had to be divorced so the stricken wife could qualify for Medicaid.

All of these dollar figures raise issues of serious concern for all of us, as health care consumers and as taxpayers. As long as hospital costs and other health care costs continue to rise at such a rapid rate, your insurance coverage will not keep up. Consequently, if you or a member of your family are hospitalized, you will in all probability end up paying far more out of your own pocket than you had ever expected. Unfortunately, it usually takes a hospital stint to reveal how many loopholes a person has in his or her insurance coverage.

Even if you are fortunate enough never to get sick or have a sick youngster, you will still face those rising health costs. Because the health insurance industry has not yet begun to seriously question the bills presented to them by hospitals, nursing homes and other providers of care, far too many health-care providers unnecessarily duplicate one another's equipment. For example, in far too many instances, we will find two or three or more hospitals in the same city with the same extraordinarily expensive coronary care equipment, when the equipment of one of them could serve the needs of the entire city.

The result, of course, is higher overhead for all these hospitals, which means higher rates for those who get sick and higher insurance premiums even if you don't get sick.

On top of higher insurance premiums, taxes also go to pay for the increased cost of Medicare and Medicaid. Having the government pay for Medicare is, of course, proper and most appropriate. However, when a few unscrupulous practitioners take advantage of the situation and overcharge elderly patients, the program and the great majority of honest practitioners as well as the taxpayers suffer. On November 19, 1973, the *New York Times* carried the following page one headline:

Medicare Held "Gold Mine" for Doctors
in Manhattan

. . .The first public disclosure by the federal government of Medicare fees charged by doctors shows that Manhattan-based physicians usually charge more — sometimes much more — for an identical service than other practitioners in the metropolitan area.

According to Carmine F. Ammirati, Vice President and Secretary of the Blue Shield unit in New York (called United Medical Service), which administers both its own insurance and the federal insurance program, Medicare has been a gold mine for doctors.

The New York doctors cited here, although a very small number, are taking advantage of a national shortage of doctors to milk the public. This is the same as oil companies raking in "windfall profits" while the nation is experiencing an energy crisis.

Let us examine the lessons we should have learned by now from Medicare. Medicare was created in 1965 as a federal health insurance program for individuals 65 and older, and buys insurance with federal tax dollars to cover this in-hospital care. A second portion of the program, which is voluntary (although almost everyone has joined), covers doctors' bills. Medicare has gone a long way toward providing more care, but has also stimulated very rapidly rising costs that people over 65 have to assume.

Unfortunately, Medicare encourages expensive hospital care while discouraging less expensive care in nursing homes or through home health services. Medicare funds are also being paid into a disjointed system that does not guarantee quality care but does ensure continually higher costs. We have had to learn the hard way that this separate categorical approach to health problems unnecessarily contributes to inflation and doesn't always return a full dollar's worth of care for a dollar spent. In fact, inflation has been so rapid that the elderly are now paying more dollars out of their own pockets for health care than they did before Medicare was adopted in

23

1965! According to a 1973 Social Security Administration report, the average elderly person's out-of-pocket health costs have increased from $234 to $276 in six years (1966-1972). At the same time, third party insurance payments for an elderly individual have climbed from $206 to $706, well over a three-fold increase in the six years. It is evident that in providing more purchasing power — without providing concurrent improvements in the delivery system — Medicare has caused an upward spiral of prices. Because of inflation, the program has not helped our senior citizens as much as it could and should.

If the consumer is to get his money's worth from health expenditures, and if the government as a consumer and guaranteeing agent of the public is to get its own money's worth, then more attention must be paid to making sure that care is comprehensive and the system of providing the care is balanced.

Merely trying to provide more facilities could lead us into the same trap. If we continued to build new beds, there would be a tendency on the part of the hospitals to want to keep them full, and this could well lead to overuse by people who didn't need such long stays but had the insurance coverage to pay for it. More beds would do nothing, of course, for those individuals who need the care but have no means of covering the cost.

A more sophisticated health facilities problem is the overuse of exotic equipment that has recently come into existence. New life-saving programs in open heart surgery in the last decade or so have led, often for prestige purposes alone, to many local community hospitals rapidly installing open-heart surgery units. In many cases, the capacity to perform operations far exceeds the need, and in some cases, the over-supply has an adverse effect upon quality. Evidence and testimony were recently presented in a northeast state that indicated four of the six hospitals doing open-heart surgery performed operations so seldom as to call their quality into doubt.

Cobalt machines used in cancer radiotherapy are another example of expensive equipment being purchased willy-nilly by hospitals. Most of the regional and state studies have shown that the machines are being utilized at 65 percent of peak efficiency. The fact that they are not being used more effectively means that an additional cost burden is being placed on all users of hospital facilities. Under the current system, it is irrelevant that the bulk of the hospital patients have no desire or need to use cobalt machines. They have to share in paying for them.

The most startling prediction for the future of health care is the cost that will be borne by the federal budget in 1980; namely, that the $30 billion federal expenditure in 1974 will grow to approximately $70 billion by 1978, according to most health experts. This projection should get all citizens, as well as lawmakers, be they for an increased federal involvement or not, to sit up and take notice. Such a drastic increase should at least get people to explore alternatives to our current health system and their effectiveness.

The amount of federal dollars being spent in health care has gone up rapidly in the past few years. The bulk of this increase has been due to Medicare and Medicaid. For budget year 1965, almost $1 billion was spent for financing health care, whereas for budget year 1974, that amount increased to almost $20 billion. This increase alone accounts for much of the wide-scale conviction on the part of government as well as consumers that something must be done quickly in the health care field.

Another major area of federal budget increase has been in providing direct health care through government programs (as determined from Medicare and Medicaid, where the government underwrites the cost of care). The government provides direct medical services for certain special categories of beneficiaries — such as armed forces personnel and their dependents, veterans, and American Indians. Overall, the federal budget has gone from $2 billion for direct health care in 1965 to $4.5 billion in budget year 1974. This is another reason why health care has become such a pressing issue for the government and why we must do something in the very near future. The total amount of federal dollars to be spent for medical and health-related activities in budget year 1974 is $30.3 billion. The portion of that expenditure for providing hospital and medical services, either through the direct care program or indirectly through the financing programs of Medicare and Medicaid, is $24.2 billion.

Eighty cents of every federal health dollar goes to programs of care. This means that there has not been enough balance or attention paid to the other areas of the health care picture. It is ironic and indeed incomprehensible that the current administration has not seen fit to recommend a more balanced approach, but has in fact proposed to make the situation worse. Because many of the medical service programs cannot be controlled, the administration has tried to keep overall health expenditures down by eliminating programs in areas where the costs can be controlled. If this were taken to its ultimate conclusion, we would have a health policy that would pay only for health services and we would not have any program in areas such as health research and health training. Since the federal government is the only organization that can guarantee that we pursue much needed health research and help provide the necessary people to carry this on, it becomes clear that the Nixon Administration's health policy makes absolutely no sense at all.

For example, in the area of medical research, the administration proposes that there only be emphasis on a few specific diseases and this will be at the expense of more basic research. Professor Rashi Fein, a well-known economist on the Harvard University faculty, addressed this point in November 1973, at the American Public Health Association Conference. He indicated that these policies certainly did not make sense from a humanitarian standpoint. Dr. Fein stated:

> If the need of short-run economic policy is the causal factor (decline in support for a variety of health research eduational and training activities), we have every reason to be disturbed at the selection of programs that must bear the costs of the anti-inflationary drive. In

research and training programs, we are dealing with activities that, unlike construction and highway development, cannot be turned off and on without major dislocations, difficulties, wastage, and unfavorable long-term impact. Required lead-times are such that these programs will be far less productive if their levels of support fluctuate around a given average than would be the case if they were maintained at the particular average level.

If one tries to analyze the specific cuts in research, the situation becomes more absurd. The bulk of medical research in this country is done through the National Institutes of Health and its divisions, such as the National Cancer Institute and the National Institute for General Medical Sciences. The administration proposal for budget year 1974 calls for several of the institutes either to remain stagnant or to retrench in their activities. The irony of the situation is that the retrenchments are being called for in some of the very areas that the government and consumer health costs are rising most rapidly. One example is kidney research.

The federal government underwrites payment for health services through the Social Security program. It is through this program that a commitment was made to help pay the bills of those unfortunate individuals suffering from end-stage kidney disease. This program will cost close to $250 million this year, rising to approximately $1 billion in the next three or so years. The only chance we have for reducing this program's cost is to promote basic research into kidney diseases in order some day to more effectively control or eliminate them. As incredible as it seems, the budget proposed by the Nixon Administration for 1974 calls for reducing kidney research from $17 million to $15 million. If ever there was an example of being penny-wise and pound-foolish, this is it.

An alternative to increasing money for basic research on kidney disease is just to let people die. I still shudder every time I think of the situation that arose at the University of Washington.

Because we in the State of Washington have been for-

27

tunate enough to have one of the most eminent specialists in the world, Dr. Belding Scribner, working on kidney dialysis problems, the matter of determining who will live and who will die hit Washington State before the federal program was enacted. The only solution to this problem as recently as 1972 was to establish a committee that would vote to handle certain cases and not to handle others. Of course, the committee knew that not handling a certain case meant a death sentence.

Congress has now voted to include coverage of end-stage kidney disease under the Social Security program. But this program will be extraordinarily expensive unless there are research breakthroughs. My view is that government would be remiss not to invest in suitable investigations of the causes and ultimately the cures for kidney disease.

Kidney research is only one of several research areas that were recommended for leveling off by the Nixon Administration. Besides research, cutbacks were proposed for health education, organization of health care, and health care delivery. It would seem that, if we as a nation are ever going to reverse or slow down the runaway inflation in health care, the only approach is systematic long-term improvements such as curing major diseases through research.

One of the causes of skyrocketing health costs is the inadequate supply of trained health manpower. Unless we have more doctors, dentists, nurses, public health specialists and other allied health personnel, there will continue to be a demand for services that exceeds the supply of people who can give them. Hence, prices will continue to go up. Yet the administration's proposed budgets for 1974 and 1975 call for substantial decreases in support leading to the production of more health professionals. For example, it was proposed that, for the various programs in allied health (in 1973 $34 million was requested), the budget request for 1974 be completely eliminated. Yet we all know the reliance that modern-day medicine has on people such as x-ray technologists, inhalation therapists, and medical technicians. It is absurd to cut off the supply of these health practitioners. Dr. Fein has an interesting explanation for this behavior. Since he concludes that the administration has not cut research and training programs because of budget policy reasons, he then asks what possible explanation there is for cutting back in these human resources areas. He comes to the conclusion that these are merely first steps in a systematic policy that would bring about even further cuts in the future.

This budget expresses an assessment by the administration that a good deal of the federal activity in the health field should be supported by other sources. This would presumably mean by other levels of government or by the users of the programs in some kind of supply and demand economic marketplace.

If Dr. Fein's analysis of the budget is correct, then it becomes clear that the Nixon Administration budget is a political policy document. The philosophy behind it is that all attempts will be made to decrease the government funding that goes into health and medical care. This is irresponsible, because it ignores the potential benefits which come from such programs, and further ignores the likelihood that there may be no alternative ways of paying for these programs. A proposal of this sort does not for a moment take into consideration the most likely future course of events, namely, that if areas such as research and training are cut back, they may be totally eliminated by our society.

Research and training are not the only areas that would be so affected. The National Academy of Sciences, through its Institute of Medicine, did an analysis of the administration's health budget. They found that, excluding Medicare and Medicaid, the President's 1974 budget recommended that health programs be reduced by $52.2 million below the 1973 level. These reductions included $17 million from the Food and Drug Administration, $5 million from the Indian health programs, $70 million from mental health programs, and even $17 million from preventive health programs such as lead-base paint poison prevention and rat control. This is in addition to two major reductions of $150 million for planning and development activities and almost $300 million in manpower training programs for doctors, nurses, and other health professionals. Reductions this expansive and this deep in so many important aspects of the government's activities in health can lead to only one conclusion: that there is a systematic and short-sighted attempt on the part of the current administration to steer away from the areas that will lead to a long-term program and future improvements in health care. This would affect our efforts to set standards of care, to keep the environment livable and safe, and to provide sufficient resources to allow everyone to get care without causing rampant inflation. Suffice it to say at this point that the fundamental issue has been raised through the proposed cutbacks in health areas. It becomes very important, then, to realize what the impact of such proposals will be if carried out.

Looking at several of the proposed reductions should be sufficient to convince anyone not only that these programs are important in the national interest and therefore should be funded by the federal government, but also that there is no other readily available source of funds to pick up the slack if the federal government withdraws from its commitment.

One area, for example, is preventive health and communicable diseases. These diseases are reduced by immunization and treatment when necessary. The role of the government has been to prevent diseases through research, and provide services and public information. Its activities include immunization, laboratory improvements, and control of diseases that get transmitted through migration borders.

Only a few years ago, Americans could congratulate themselves for chasing the spectre of epidemic disease from the nation's cribs and schoolyards.

So writes Patricia F. Bode in the *National Observer*, August 25, 1973. Immunization against polio, diphtheria, whooping cough, and other contagious diseases reached an all-time high.

But officials at the United States Center for Disease Control say that surveys show that approximately five million of the nation's one-to-four-year-old children are insufficiently immunized. Health experts now warn that complacency has taken over. Parents have allowed immunization levels to drop at an alarming rate. Of the 14 million pre-school children in this country, one out of every three is insufficiently immunized.

Thus far, the result of this inadequate protection of our children has not proved to be a public health disaster. However, it is inexcusable that approximately 50 children died and more than 40,000 youngsters developed complications including brain damage due to measles last year.

One of the greatest success stories in American medicine has been the determination of the causes and the development of immunization by vaccination — a very inexpensive and easy cure for polio. Surveys now indicate, however, that in 1964, 88 percent of American pre-schoolers were protected against polio. This figure dropped to 63 percent in 1973. The figure is even lower (51 percent) for non-white pre-school children living in the central cities of major metropolitan areas.

The problem is even greater than the danger of isolated cases, according to Dr. John J. Witte, chief of the Center for Disease Control, Immunization Branch. He says that the existence of five million pre-schoolers means epidemics are quite possible:

We have every reason to believe that polio could spread significantly if introduced in certain areas.

It is impossible to increase attention to the need for immunizing pre-schoolers when the Administration proposes to cut back on its programs.

In addition to the control of communicable diseases, emphasis must be placed on drug abuse problems, mental illness, crime prevention, venereal disease, and special health problems for certain areas of the country such as black lung disease.

A second area worth noting is environmental health problems. These programs are devised to control such problems as lead-base paint poisoning and rats, two health hazards most prevalent in lower income neighborhoods.

The federal government is empowered to come up with environmental standards and serve as a watchdog to make sure that these standards are obeyed. It would seem downright foolish to cut back on these programs. The future of our nation, particularly the current generation of children, would suffer tremendously if we cut back on the relatively small amount of money that is currently being spent in controlling lead poisoning and rats.

Another major area to consider is that of consumer protection. The federal programs here are designed to protect the public from impure foods, unsafe and ineffective drugs and hazardous consumer products. The Food and Drug Administration (FDA), another unit of HEW, plays an important role in improving the quality and safety of the nation's food supply and the safety and effectiveness of drugs for their intended uses. They are also responsible for reviewing the usefulness of vaccinations and are required to conduct inspections of blood banks. The consumer needs more protection in these areas, not less. It is difficult if not impossible to see how anyone would pick up the slack in these program areas if the federal government pulled back.

Congress recently identified another important area to stress in the future by passing my bill to establish a Consumer Product Safety Commission. The commission will conduct investigations, and research, collect and make available information to protect the consumer from hazardous products and to inform the public about the safe use of those which are potentially hazardous if not handled properly.

Another example is the problem of accidents and occupational health. In 1971 there were 155,000 accidental deaths. Furthermore, accidents are the leading cause of death for persons aged 1 to 37. If these statistics are not horrendous enough, it should be noted that more than eleven million people (one out of every twenty Americans) were disabled during 1971 as a result of accidents. Approximately 55,000 deaths were the result of traffic accidents. This clearly suggests a need for increasing rather than cutting back on our highway safety program, and this is also true for occupational safety and health. All of these are public health programs and should be supported by the public. There does not seem to be anyone likely to pick up any cutbacks by the federal government, nor does there appear to be any good reason why this should be done. Federal programs also support community health care facilities which serve the general public, as well as facilities operated by federal agencies for the special groups for which the government provides care.

The federal program supporting community health care facilities (the Hill-Burton program in HEW) has become still another major source of policy dispute. To take the position that the government should underwrite health facilities does not mean that the nation needs a large new supply of hospital beds. Nationwide there may be an oversupply of hospital beds, and further, the occupancy rate in hospitals has been declining since 1969. But the fact remains that there are pockets of the country that need more beds than they currently have, a reflection of population shifts. In addition, there are hospitals in many areas, particularly in older inner-city urban areas, that require the replacement of beds and equipment that have become obsolete. There also is a need to redirect construction of community health care facilities away from in-patient facilities in order to provide more out-patient facilities. It is foolhardy to suggest, as the current administration has, that the hospital facilities program (the Hill-Burton) is not needed. If we are to succeed in improving care, then such a program is essential and the government must underwrite it.

The final area that deserves attention at the highest levels is the organization and delivery of health services. A prime concern must be the regional medical program, geared toward delivering the latest in health technology to victims of heart disease, stroke, and cancer. The program focuses upon the delivery and organization of health services and the long-term role of the federal government. If the federal government is only to engage in research that is focused on improving the delivery of care (as the current administration proposes), then the nagging question is: who will provide the money to develop the technology and care for patients once the research has shown the best way to proceed? Short of any other source, we must all assume that this is an appropriate role for the federal government.

It may be useful in summarizing the role of the federal government in health care to look at two reports done in 1968 and 1970, respectively, by the Senate Committee on Government Operations. The subcommittee studying these areas was under the chairmanship of Senator Abraham Ribicoff, a former Secretary of Health, Education, and Welfare. The committee, after long study, concluded that:

> The nation's private health care system was on the verge of crisis: large numbers of poor received improper care or no care at all; the middle class felt the financial pressure of the high cost of care and lived in fear of prolonged and expensive catastrophic illness; the care both received often was fragmented and impersonal.

The report then went on to indicate that health insurance plans, by generally covering only care administered in hospitals, encouraged the most expensive care possible. In addition, by covering treatment instead of prevention, the plans were paying for sickness more than health.

With respect to health services and health manpower, programs had failed to keep pace with advances in medical science and changes in society. They appeared to be organized more for the convenience and concern of their practitioners and institutions than for the health needs and financial security of the patient.

It is difficult to point out what improvements subsequent to the 1970 report have made these statements any less applicable today.

3. Priorities and Directions

The following examples of children's safety, diseases, and environmental hazards serve to point out how difficult it is to make priority choices. It is clear to me that we are not moving fast enough in many areas of human health, safety, and protection. Citizen protection must be balanced with other demands on our limited resources. But just as society has determined that public school education is a long-term investment that should receive public funds, so too should health care and public protection. If we need to develop these new programs by cutting back in other areas, then this should be done.

The office of the medical examiner of Dade County, Florida, wrote to the National Commission on Product Safety (1969):

> We have been reviewing the files of the Medical Examiner's office since 1956 to the present time and have found eleven cases of infant deaths due to accidental suffocation, strangulation or hanging in cribs, playpens, or car beds. The enclosed includes summaries of these eleven cases. The ages range from two months to twenty-four months, with a mean of nine months. Five of the eleven were six months of age or younger. Eight were male, and three female.

Selected Examples:

> Case 1-65-2220. This crib was a Kiddie-Coop in good repair. The crib has a top covering hinged on one side. A nine month old infant pulled himself to a standing

position, pushed up the top with his head, put his chin over the top rail of the crib, and with the crib top resting on the back of the head, pressure was applied to the neck. Apparently, he did not have the strength to free himself from this position.

Case 2-62-786. This Crib was of the regular vertical bar type. It was defective in that one corner had become unbolted. The child slipped down between the side wall and the mattress, catching his chin on the spring, and he was found hanging in this position.

Case 5-68-871. The crib was of the usual vertical bar type. One bolt was missing from the tope of one corner. A twenty month old child pushed his body through the space between the sides and the end of the crib, but the head was caught inside the crib, and he was found hanging from the corner of the crib.

The remaining eight cases are no less gruesome. The coroner's office considered the question of faulty material design in six of the eight cases. The coroner's office recommended that, if vertical bars were used in cribs, they should be sufficiently close together so that hips, abdomen and chest of the child cannot wiggle between them. Among the other recommendations were alterations in the nut and bolt construction of the sides and ends of the crib, and greater public awareness of the potential dangers of cribs repaired with wire or twine and the top covers of cribs, handles on car beds and ornamental toys for the neck of a small child.

Congress felt that the protection of the public demanded that infant furniture and other items such as household chemicals and toys meet sufficient standards to indeed protect the consumer; hence, the establishment of a Consumer Product Safety Commission. Priorities in this country should be such that the public is guaranteed that harmless-looking children's furniture should not be potential death traps.

Sudden Infant Death Syndrome (SIDS) is the leading cause of death in the United States among infants between one month and one year of life. Yet, why these babies die is unknown.

The shock, anguish and guilt of the parents in these situations is incredible. The letters reprinted in this book from unfortunate parents can express these feelings far better than anyone could describe. SIDS, of course, is illustrative of several equally agonizing childhood diseases. Muscular dystrophy, genetic diseases such as Cooley's Anemia, hemophilia, Tay-Sachs, cerebral palsy, mental illness and others also require more understanding so that better treatments can be uncovered.

And yet, on June 20, 1973, the administration sent Dr. Gerald D. LaVeck to represent them in proposing a cutback in research grants for this problem. It should be pointed out that this was Dr. LaVeck's last hearing as a government representative. Ten days later, on the first of July, he quit the administration to return to the medical center at the University of Washington in Seattle.

I cannot help but include an aside at this point. One of the greatest shames of all that has come about because of the severe cutbacks in health by the Nixon Administration has been this: it has driven out of government service some of the finest health professionals in the country. Distinguished scientists and scholars, such as Surgeon General Jesse Steinfeld, National Institutes of Health Director Robert Marston and Deputy Director Robert Berliner, and Director of Child Health and Human Development LaVeck have all been driven out of government by a hostile administration.

On January 16, 1974, Dr. John Sherman, Deputy Director of NIH, was added to the list. He quit because he was "discouraged and disillusioned," adding that "what is at stake is the essence of this place." Sherman, who joined NIH in 1953 as a research pharmacologist, spoke nostalgically of the pride which he said every administration except this one had taken in the agency's worldwide reputation for excellence. "John Gardner," he recalled, "used to refer to the NIH as one of the jewels in the crown of HEW when he was secretary of the department (during the Johnson Administration). But that positive attitude is missing now."

The fact that, over the years, the advances in health and

37

medical science have been completely bipartisan is illustrated by a June 20 hearing before the Senate Appropriations Subcommittee on Health, by the distinguished Republican Senator from New Hampshire, Norris Cotton. Senator Cotton is the ranking Republican member of the subcommittee, and has served the State of New Hampshire and the nation in a selfless and extraordinary fashion for several years. One of the happiest feelings I had in receiving the Lasker Award was the fact that Senator Cotton, at great personal inconvenience, flew cross-country to speak at Seattle at the dinner and share in the award on behalf of the entire U.S. Senate.

Senator Cotton: You say the Institute (referring to the Institute of Child Health and Human Development) will increase its program on sudden infant death, yet you are cutting down on research grants for this problem.

Dr. LaVeck: In 1974, we plan to spend about $3.5 million on the sudden infant death syndrome. This is the amount we will be spending also in 1973, the current year. And in 1972 there was approximately the same amount, about $3.5 million. We have had little change in the total amount of money available for sudden infant deaths in the past three years.

Dr. LaVeck cannot answer directly the probing question of Senator Cotton, because the answer is that the institute would have to cut down on research grants for this problem because of already outstanding commitments. This vague answer is not Dr. LaVeck's fault. Administration witnesses have been carefully coached and prompted before they can testify on Capitol Hill.

Possible answers are now emerging as to causes of the sudden infant death syndrome. One possibility being examined is that death is caused by poor nervous system control over heart and lung functions during sleep. Institute research showed that these deaths are handled with varying degrees of knowledge and understanding, and that the families of victims may be poorly dealt with by professionals, the community, and relatives. The Institute needs to increase its basic research and it also needs to increase its programs of public and professional education, in order to resolve these problems and encourage more scientists to study the syndrome. Progress cannot come through reducing the number of research grants to study the problem.

The Washington Post reported (January 9, 1974) that: "More than a third of about 6,000 youngsters (in Milwaukee, Wisconsin) living in a 25-square block area of the inner city here have been found to be suffering from some degree of lead poisoning."

Of 6,626 children under the age of six tested between July 1972 and September of last year, 2,343 children; or 35 percent, were found to have "potentially dangerous" levels of lead in their body. Almost all the children had to undergo immediate treatment, taking medication that caused them to excrete the excess lead. About a dozen of the children had to be hospitalized for treatment. There were no deaths. The 34 percent figure is one of the highest found in the United States. A U.S. Public Health Service survey in 27 cities in 1971 found an average rate of lead poisoning among inner city youngsters to be 21 percent.

The Milwaukee results came from the first year of a three-year $230,000 federally funded city campaign against lead poisoning.

A total of $15 million was requested for the Public Health Service (PHS) for lead poisoning campaigns in cities in the six-state Midwest region of Wisconsin, Illinois, Ohio, Indiana, Michigan and Minnesota. However, PHS allotted only $1.5 million to such campaigns.

Roughly 60 percent of the youngsters found with 40 micrograms of lead per millileter of blood or higher were less than 3½ years old.

City health officials surmised that the most frequent cause of the poisoning was eating paint chips or plaster containing lead. Poisoning was more frequent in the poor areas, it was felt, because more homes were dilapidated with peeling paint and plaster. It was further compounded among the young, officials said, by a malady of unknown cause called pica, a compulsion among some children to eat non-food items such as paint, plaster, rags, newspapers, magazines or dirt.

When not treated in its earliest stages, lead poisoning can cause damage to the brain and nervous system resulting in permanent loss of muscle control, mental retardation or blindness.

The protection of the public demands that the environment for children be sufficiently lead-free to protect our youngsters from brain damage, mental retardation, blindness, and even death.

It is a legitimate concern of government to worry about all human protection areas, including the protection of children. We, of course, have to strike a balance among all our concerns. But when we are dealing with the very life and death of our citizens, and we know how to save lives, we should do it.

During 1973, the General Accounting Office (GAO) helped Senator Mansfield and me to uncover the fact that $140 million was being impounded (not spent) by the Nixon Administration on medical research. This money was slated to go to cancer research. And, as incredible as it seems, the same amount of money ($140 million) was being spent on secret raids in Cambodia. These bombings were not made known to either the public or to Congress. This is to me certainly a case of misplaced priorities. An undeclared and unwinnable war in Cambodia was getting money over a winnable war against cancer.

There is no doubt that in the long run the investment that we make in the health area will be recovered. A healthier population will be more productive. People who are currently supported by public welfare and public funds will be replaced by people who will be earning money in useful jobs and will be paying taxes.

Polio is a good example. By cutting death and disability because of polio, we have saved thousands of individuals who would otherwise be crippled, not working, and having to be supported for medical care as well as for the other basics of life. The miracles of science have solved this problem through a simple vaccine.

Dr. Lewis Thomas, currently the President of Memorial Sloan Kettering Cancer Center, provided us with this kind of hope for all diseases. Appearing before the Senate Health Appropriations Subcommittee in February 1973, he indicated:

> . . . that most if not all of the major human diseases represent approachable scientific problems, open to solution sooner or later. . . I have no more difficulty in imagining a human community free of disease than I do in envisioning healthy plants or healthy stocks of valuable animals.

This country has long guaranteed its citizens the right to public education. Health care should also be a right guaranteed by government.

Having proposed that health care is a right to be enjoyed by all our citizens, the harder problem then lies ahead: how to move from where we are now to the goal, particularly within a short period of time. This does not mean that all disease will be eliminated by a certain date; that may take decades. What it does mean, however, is that all health consumers should have the best care available to them when they need it.

In determining priorities and directions, we must recognize that there have been major changes in the medical care needs of our citizens in the past few decades. The overriding change has been the dramatic decrease in diseases that can be classified as acute or infectious, and a shift to long-term chronic diseases. Major killers of the past were diseases such as smallpox, cholera, diphtheria, typhoid, and bubonic plague. In addition, pneumonia, tuberculosis, and diarrhea were major causes of death and are now relatively rare. These diseases have been replaced by a new set. Heart disease, stroke, and cancer are the top three causes of death currently. These diseases are more difficult to diagnose, take longer to treat, and are much more expensive.

It is important to take into consideration the differences

41

associated with the major killers of today. They are generally diseases which last a long time; they are due to wearing-out of certain parts of the body and are degenerative in nature, often coming about as a result of many different causes and requiring different types of treatments.

One of the ways to direct health care priorities is to view the system from the vantage point of the health consumer. From that perspective, many things fall into place more easily. For example, medical research which takes into account the needs of the public must include applying the latest techniques for medical knowledge to people suffering from disease. This statement is not meant to stir up the age-old debate within the science community about more basic research vs. more applied research. Rather, it makes the case that we may have to determine the working of the cell or parts of the cell before we can cure even some types of cancer. However, it may be possible to control certain types without that basic knowledge. We have a good number of examples to illustrate both approaches.

Research Priorities

A classical example of this conflict is the Salk vaccine, which was used as an interim measure against polio, and is a story validly described in Steven Strickland's book, *Politics, Science, and Dread Disease.* It was clear at the time that Sabin's much-improved vaccine was on the way. The national foundation which released the Salk vaccine defined its position by stating that they were able to have Salk's vaccine on the market five years before the Sabin formula was ready for distribution.

Interim steps like the Salk vaccine can be very expensive; but who is to say that countless thousands of Americans who are walking around today and functioning perfectly might not have been among those who came down with polio during the years that the Salk vaccine was available and the Sabin was not?

The *New York Times,* in a 1966 editorial, addressed this very point. It declared that it was a mistake to wait before we acted until almost total knowledge is available. As an example, Edward Jenner did not know of the germ theory of disease or the viral origin of smallpox, but introduced a smallpox vaccination more than 150 years ago which has left us scarcely aware of what smallpox is, let alone the death and disability it can produce.

Strickland's book tells the story of Senator Lister Hill's fight to bring the latest medical achievements to the public. Senator Hill was a stalwart of the Senate, one of my predecessors as Chairman of the Appropriations Health Subcommittee, and one of the greatest proponents of health research this country has ever seen. The story includes a dialogue between Dr. Irving Wright and Senator Hill in 1956, describing a medical breakthrough made in spite of the skepticism of many so-called experts at that time.

Dr. Wright: We therefore started to treat a series of patients suffering from coronary thrombosis with anticoagulant therapy. This was in 1942.

Senator Hill: That was pioneering, so to speak.

Dr. Wright: That is right, and it was looked on by us as a pilot stody.

Senator Hill: And I suppose you met great resistance, did you not?

Dr. Wright: Great resistance.

Senator Hill: That is the usual story, is it not?

Dr. Wright: At first, they say 'It couldn't be so,' and later, 'We knew it all the time.'

Priorities should be set with an eye to the future. Experts tell us that 85 percent or so of those who will be sick in the 1970's could be cared for by a general practitioner or a physician assistant or nurse practitioner without being hospitalized. There appears to be a need for continuous care under the supervision of some broadly-trained health practitioner. The modern "epidemics" of cancer, heart disease, arthritis, mental illness, industrial diseases, accidents, and so on, present a more complex task than in the past.

Diseases appear to have multiple causes, including genetic, environmental, and social factors. Smoking, over-eating, overdrinking, and lack of exercise are patterns of behavior that seem to contribute to the onset and severity of certain diseases.

With this complex series of chronic diseases staring us in the face, we must begin to concentrate more on the prevention and protection side of the health care equation. Not only is this a much more inexpensive way of dealing with our problems, but also a number of people may not know that they have a predisposition to a disease, or are unaware that medical intervention at a certain point might save their lives. Third, people have little control over the air they breath, water they drink, food they eat, and manufacturing of cars they buy or clothes they wear. Government is the only entity that can handle these problems. We must concentrate more on screening for certain kinds of diseases, and pay much more at-tention to the environmental hazards of our industrialized society.

One important consideration would be what happens if we continue with only the existing health legislation, putting more and more government dollars into personal health ser-vices, the bulk of these dollars going into direct treatment. This is obviously the costliest way we can use our health dollars. For example, in 1966, 6 percent of all of our nation's dollars (termed the Gross National Product) were going into health care. This amounted to $212 per person. In 1974, the percentage of the Gross National Product in health is estimated at 7.7 percent and will amount to $440 per person. If the future trends continue, and every indication seems to be that they will, the $800 per person we will spend by the year 1980 will represent about 10 percent of the Gross National Product.

To look at this in positive terms and try to reset priorities, we might be able to do as follows. If Congress and the public are convinced that, in the year 1980, we would be spending close to $80 billion federal money for health just by continuing with the current legislation (we are currently spending approximately $33 billion for health), we should then be able to make a compelling case to spend the same $80 billion to become more efficient and concentrate on preventing accidents, lowering environmental risks, encouraging new scientific breakthroughs, and getting needed care to people in a more timely fashion.

To use the example that has been cited often in this book, namely kidney disease research, it could be pointed out that if we only continue with the current legislation whereby the government pays for end-stage renal disease, then the cost to the government in 1980 will be approximately $3 billion. However, if we chose to triple or even quadruple our investment in kidney disease research and technology, the research costs still would amount to $60 million a year. It is entirely possible that this kind of investment in the prevention and control side of our health care system might very well lead to breakthroughs that would cut down substantially on an expenditure which is fifty times as great.

Since we are already committed to including care for end-stage kidney disease in the Social Security program, it would seem that even the most hard-headed businessman would think that it is a good investment for our nation to triple or quadruple the investment in kidney research.

This example should help to point out that just putting more money into the health system may not be enough. We should make important changes in the priorities and directions now.

By doing this, the government can really help the individual consumer to be on surer footing. It would allow for protection against situations where unexpected accidents or illnesses might wipe out a family's finances. This protection must come in two situations: first, to insure care in case of unexpected illness, and second, to put brakes on the present rapid inflation, where the same dollar buys less care.

For the unexpected illness or accident, particularly the expensive one, there must be adequate health insurance. The best situation would be to know, just as you now know how much it costs for a month or a year of automobile insurance or household theft insurance, that you have a health insurance policy that will cover your health care needs. This will be discussed in greater detail in the chapter on health financing.

Choices are not very easy. Dr. Kerr White, in his *Scientific American* article, "Life and Death in Medicine," describes some of these difficult priority choices:

What social or even medical utility is to be accorded diagnostic ability if it is not accompanied by effective action and an acceptable outcome? Because we have mastered some procedure, does it follow that society should make it available to all who seek it? To all who can pay for it? To all who need it? Is the new procedure to be preferred over some other form of intervention for the same health problem?

For example, should we concentrate on perfecting coronary artery by-pass operations, or on improving early detection and better management for patients with coronary artery insufficiency? Should we concentrate on dialysis and transplants for chronic kidney disease or on early detection, coordinated medical management, and follow-up of initial urinary tract infections? In short, should we continue to develop and rely heavily on complex medical technology for the treatment of acute or life-threatening diseases and conditions? Or would we be better advised to broaden our approach and devote more of our efforts to identifying, containing, or resolving the health problems that have major impacts on the quality of our lives?

Should resources currently expended on pills, potions and procedures whose benefit or efficacy have never been objectively evaluated be shifted to the provision of personnel and services to make living with chronic disability more comfortable and dying more dignified? How much responsibility has medicine for the terminally ill? What are the limits of these responsibilities and who decides? Are the decisions determined by scientific knowledge and available technology, or by ethical, social and humanitarian considerations, or by a mixture of both? Is it enough to tell the patient that he has chronic heart failure and prescribe a suitable regimen, or should he and his family be taught to manage the problem so that he can live a satisfying life within the limits of his own capacity, without restricting unduly the rights and independence of his family and his community? To what extent should the doctor be responsible for educating his community so that its members can better cope with current epidemics of accidents, alcoholism, delinquency, drug dependence, deprivation, inadequate parenting, loneliness, occupational boredom, and suicide?

These are the questions that we must deal with during the 1970s and beyond.

If you or a member of your family are a victim of a heart condition or kidney disease as described by Dr. White, you know the answer to the questions that are posed. The problem to you is too personal to be presented as an abstract choice. If the technology is available, then you want to receive that kind of operation or care, particularly if it is a matter of life or death. Long-term preventive care and improvement for the next generation and society at large are too abstract to be dealt with under this set of circumstances.

But, if we are to improve society and make life more enjoyable, safer, and healthier in the future, then we must do both — provide the necessary research and the preventive care and consumer education — to guarantee our citizens better care tomorrow while we do all we can for those who are sick today.

This discussion of priorities sets the stage for the next three chapters. These case studies are examples of congressional action to help focus priorities. Chapter Four presents the discussion of a large scale infusion of new resources into conquering cancer. Chapter Five discusses a series of governmental thrusts to protect consumers, and Chapter Six focuses upon a specific need for accident prevention through the creation of a product safety commission.

4.   The Conquest of Cancer

Some people see things as they are and ask why: I
dream dreams that never were and ask why not.

George Bernard Shaw

These words could well be used as the rallying cry for
eliminating cancer within our lifetime.

This country took a major step toward that goal when on
December 23, 1971, the National Cancer Act was signed into
law in the White House, witnessed by leading cancer researchers and administrators and a number of fellow Senators
and Congressmen who had seen the bill through its passage in
the House and Senate.

President Nixon inaugurated this new era of expanded
cancer effort with what he called ". . . a total commitment of
Congress and the President . . . to provide the funds for the
conquest of cancer." The President declared: "We must put
our money where our hopes are in finding a cancer cure."

The legislation set up a three-man Cancer Panel to
monitor the program. Chosen to be Chairman was Benno C.
Schmidt, a businessman with considerable background and
experience in the management of cancer research. He is the
chairman of Memorial Sloan Kettering Cancer Center in New
York and also served as the chairman of the National Panel of
Consultants on the Conquest of Cancer.

One of the most important features of the National Can-

49

cer Act was its large commitment of financial resources. Authorization levels were set at $420, $530, and $640 million for fiscal years 1972, 1973, and 1974 respectively.

The partnership between Congress and the President, the "total commitment" to conquer cancer, was well on the way — or so it seemed. Less than two years after the signing of the bill, the cancer program has turned into a cruel hoax. Rather than provide the funds, as President Nixon said he would in December 1971, the Administration froze and impounded $60 million in cancer research funds in 1973.

The situation became so bad that President Nixon's appointed Chairman, Benno Schmidt, declared publicly that the Administration's research policies were harming the cancer effort.

In a December 1973 speech, Schmidt noted that "neither the cancer program nor bio-medical research can thrive" if the budget for basic research continues to suffer funding cutbacks.

Science (December 1973) quoted Schmidt as follows:

"Despite expressions to the contrary by the assistant secretary for health, it is my opinion that the National Cancer Act of 1971 is a sound piece of legislation that has worked extremely well," he told a crowd of physicians attending the National Conference on Virology and Immunology in Human Cancer, held recently in New York. The mistakes that have been made, in his opinion, should be blamed on the Administration, not the cancer legislation. Schmidt thinks it was a mistake for the Administration to cut research training grants and to reduce funds for other areas of research at a time when progress in cancer depends upon progress in other areas as well. "At the time we were urging on Congress and the Administration a greater effort in cancer, we were very explicit in the position that the increased cancer effort should not be at the expense of other bio-medical research. I must confess that I, for one, did not believe that would happen." Now, Schmidt admits that he was wrong.

Dr. James D. Watson, Nobel laureate and member of the National Cancer Advisory Board, told a Maryland reporter on December 20, 1973: "The net effect of the various executive mandates over the past few months has been to decrease money going toward basic biological research."

Congress remains committed in its enthusiasm for an assault on cancer. My Senate Appropriations Subcommittee, in its report on the HEW appropriations bill for Fiscal Year 1974, indicated that:

The Committee remains steadfast in its commitment to heart and cancer research, but refuses to take part in wholesale trade-offs where human life is involved.

Cancer is a terribly complicated subject. It is not a single disease, and probably won't lend itself to a single cure. It is many diseases, and many approaches will be required. Progress will come on them one by one, unless we have a miraculous cure, which none of us truly expects today.

In April 1971, Congress received the report on the National Panel of Consultants on the Conquest of Cancer. The Panel, chaired by Benno C. Schmidt, with Dr. Sidney Farber as Co-Chairman, and Dr. William B. Hutchinson from the cancer center in my hometown, Seattle, found that cancer is the number one health concern of the American people. A poll conducted in 1966 showed that 62 percent of the public feared cancer more than any other disease. Of the 200 million Americans alive today, 50 million will develop cancer at present rates of incidence, and 34 million will die of this painful disease if better methods of prevention and treatment are not discovered.

This report was a call for action and Congress translated it into the National Cancer Act. It was not the first call for government action. As long ago as 1928, in a speech on the floor of the Senate, the senior Senator from West Virginia, Matthew M. Neely, passionately described the horrors of cancer:

> Mr. President, the concluding chapter of a *Tale of Two Cities* contains a vivid description of the guillotine, the most efficacious mechanical destroyer of human life that brutal and bloodthirsty man has ever invented.
>
> But through all the years, the victims of the guillotine have been limited to a few hundred thousand of the people of France.
>
> I propose to speak of a monster that is more insatiable than the guillotine; more destructive to life and health and happiness than the World War; more irresistible than the mightiest army that ever marched to the battle; more terrifying than any other scourge that has ever threatened the existence of the human race. The monster of which I speak has infested, and still infests, every inhabited country; it has preyed, and still preys, upon every nation; it has fed and feasted and fattened . . . on the flesh and blood and brains and bones of men and women and children in every land; the sighs and sobs and shrieks that it has exhorted from the perishing humanity would, if they were tangible things, make a mountain. The tears, which it has wrung from weeping women's eyes would make an ocean. The blood which it has shed would redden every wave that rolls on every sea. The name of this loathsome, deadly, and insatiate monster is cancer.

Stephen P. Strickland begins his fine book, *Politics, Science, and Dread Disease,* with this speech by Senator Neely. He then goes on to describe the Senator's call for government action. Neely introduced a bill which would provide a $5 million reward "to the first person who discovered a practical and successful cure for cancer."

It is sad that a cancer cure could not have been found so easily. We would have saved not only many millions of dollars, but prevented incalculable pain and suffering as well.

Since the impassioned speech by Senator Neely in 1928, we have spent over $2 billion in cancer research and have learned that the problem is much more complex than could possibly have been envisioned at that time. But many people can be treated and indeed, in some cases, cured from cancers which were fatal only a few years ago. Still, many cancers remain both totally fatal and unresponsible to any treatment at this time. A last point worth mentioning is that many unfortunate victims of cancer are being "taken" by promises of cures which do not exist, and by enrolling in insurance policies which sound good but afford them no real protection from the financial burden of this awful disease.

We obviously do not know how we will conquer all aspects of this disease. But we no longer argue whether curing cancer is an appropriate federal role. The point of dispute is over the priority it deserves.

It was a decade after Senator Neely's proposal that a cancer institute was created by the federal government. It gives me a good deal of pride to recall that the author of the bill was Senator Homer T. Bone from our State of Washington, and that I was the author of the bill in the House of Representatives. It is an obvious source of pride to residents of the State of Washington — particularly researchers at the University of Washington Medical Center and those of us who have watched the Fred Hutchinson Cancer Center grow—to reflect that the National Cancer Institute was conceived in both Houses of Congress by Washington State Congressional representatives. The national shame is that even now individuals like Fred Hutchinson, the great baseball pitcher and manager for whom the Seattle cancer center was named, are still struck down in the prime of life by cancer.

Approval of the cancer institute came by unanimous votes in both the House and the Senate. After my senior colleague, as well as my close friend, former Senator Bone, had shepherded the proposal through the Senate, we considered the passage of the bill in the House of Representatives.

It is illustrative to look back and see the arguments that I used at that time in order to pass such an important and momentous bill. One must keep in mind that this was a period when Congress paid a good deal of attention to agricultural crops and animal production.

Let word arrive at any time of a new pest attacking the fruit industry, or let a scourge of insect life invade the cotton fields, and legislatures of the state and nation stand ready to smite the rock of finance and pour forth rivers of revenue to repel the dangerous invader. Let there be news of an unknown disease of cattle and scientists march to the battlefield bulwarked with millions of good American dollars to overcome the foe. In 1936, this Congress appropriated $1,715,000 for the eradication of tuberculosis in cattle. In the same year, over half a million dollars was granted by this Congress to remove ticks from cattle, while $125,000 was employed in the destruction of the disease of hard cholera . . . I have no quarrel with the appropriation of these funds. I have no objection to the sound economic reasons behind these grants. But it is a sad commentary on our civilization when we realize that not more than $700,000 a year is spent in the entire United States on cancer research. The pitiful truth is that our national government spends only $100,000 a year on such research work.

As one can easily see, the question of choices and priorities which we currently face is not a new one. The only thing new at that time was establishing the important principle that the concern for human life was so important that our national government should become involved in it through supported research. It was of course clear that cancer was in no way a new problem. My research at that time led me to conclude the following in my address on the floor of the House:

Modern scientists know now that the Byzantine empress Theodora, wife of Justinian, the lawgiver, succumbed to a breast cancer in the year 548 A.D. Down through the centuries since man wrote his records in books, we find that phantom spectre stalking across the pages of history, leaving behind his trail of misery and pain.

54

Queen Anne, the daughter of Philip III of Spain; Mary Tudor, daughter of Henry VIII and the first of his six wives, Catherine of Aragon; the Bonapartes are further proof of the fact that cancer is no respecter of persons or personages and yet, I repeat, with all the advances made by modern science, 153,000 people a year die in the United States alone from this disease, and we in the past have been interested enough to appropriate $100,000 a year to find out what it is all about!

It is almost staggering to think about the fourteen centuries between the time of Empress Theodora and this debate on the House floor — and to think about the hundreds of thousands of people, peasants as well as kings, who have succumbed to this dread disease.

My speech on the floor in 1937 also raised the issue of consumer protection which has only recently received the important consideration it deserves in the halls of Congress. It is clear from the following paragraph that quack cancer "cures" were rampant:

Another horror which riddles our land is the cancer quack, who thrives on the ignorant and unfortunate who hope for surcease from their cancer-induced woes. This measure and the publicity being given its passage should go a long way toward convincing cancer sufferers of the necessity of early medical attention and diagnosis upon the first appearance of what might seem to be cancer symptoms. Those with lack of knowledge have been ready prey for the jackals who travel along the medical borderline. 'Benign and malignant tumors' are the distinguishing definitions used by scientists, but the quack is never benign, and his malignancy is exceeded only by his success in plying his frightful trade.

We still have a great number of quacks (with only slightly more sophisticated approaches) who are ready, willing and able to bilk the public. The best way to reduce this problem is to provide safeguards for the public and provide more education about such practices. However, until we are able to supply medical and scientific answers to people who are doomed by cancer, it will be difficult to convince some people that "miracles" might not work for them.

In 1971, when Congress passed the National Cancer Act, I still felt compelled to warn of false hopes of immediate success and simple cures in an early tomorrow. The speech in 1971 included the following:

> The problems of bio-medical science, of cancer and other dread diseases, cannot be compared with our technological problems.
>
> Our knowledge about cells and the basic building blocks of human life and even all the real functions of various organs within the human body is still too meagre. If there is a latch-key to that knowledge, it is people who are especially trained and competent in their fields of expertise who are given adequate support to probe the unknown. This takes both time and treasure, and regrettably, time cannot be simply purchased.

Time, money, and strong commitment are needed to conquer cancer. The federal government has over the past few decades shown unstinting and growing commitment to eradicating cancer. This certainly has been true of Congress. I would like to think that the cutbacks by the current Administration are merely temporary aberrations in a long-term priority of commitment. The passage of the National Cancer Act marked the first time in our history that the conquering of a disease was made a national priority. People throughout our country were finally aroused enough to convince their Congressmen that more should be done to combat this disease. This public action was important in many ways, but its main significance was to place the conquest of cancer in a new category. People expected not only their doctor but also their Congressman to do something about a specific health problem. Only a high degree of popular commitment can "land a man on the moon" in the area of public health.

In 1900, cancer was considered a completely hopeless disease. People were reluctant to talk about it. Now the attitude is much more open. Most patients want to know about their cancer and what the prognosis is. This openness has had much to do with the increasing demand by the public to get government to do something about the problem. In the 1930s, at the time the National Cancer Institute was created, scientists told us that we could save or cure twenty percent of all cancers; that is, one in five. Now they talk of saving or curing 33 percent, or one in three. If all the available techniques and information were used, that figure could be closer to 50 percent. The American Cancer Society estimates that 109,000 cancer patients will probably die in 1974 who might have been saved by earlier and better treatment. This statistic points out how much more we have to do.

We have also learned much more about the disease and the risks involved in activities such as cigarette smoking. I would like to think that cigarette labeling, which Congress passed, and my description of the hazards of cigarette tars and nicotines in my book, *Dark Side of the Marketplace* (Prentice Hall, 1968), helped bring about more public awareness.

We know that at the present time there are at least 100 different types of cancer, although we do not know the exact causes. We know that it is not contagious but that certain environmental factors such as x-rays, chemicals such as asbestos and benzidine, and other irritants lead to cancers.

We know we can do better. In 1974 there will be 75,000 deaths from lung cancer. Millions of Americans have refused to face the stark fact that they may be smoking themselves into an early grave. Also, there will be a 10 percent increase in fatalities for women in 1974, paralleling an increase in women smokers. On the positive side, in spite of a continuing increase in cigarette consumption, there has been a marked trend toward use of filter cigarettes. Twenty years ago the filter cigarette market was 3.2 percent, but has since reached 84 percent of the total. There is no doubt that this is the result of the health warnings and publicity which Congress has pushed so strenuously.

As research into cancer has become more sophisticated,

scientists have identified factors in the environment that play a role in the occurrence of cancer. This means that government must also be concerned about environmental hazards if a war on cancer is to be total.

Environmental causes of cancer are usually described in three categories: chemicals, radiation, and waste materials. Chemicals causing cancer were first discovered almost 200 years ago, in 1775, by an English surgeon who observed that chimney sweeps in England were prone to cancer of the scrotum, which was attributed to their long contact with the soot in chimneys. This was the first clear description of cancer as an occupational hazard.

Other chemicals known as hydrocarbons, which are found in polluted air and a wide variety of tars and oils, have been linked to cancer in animals. Scientists have been searching for simple relationships between chemical structure and the inducing of cancer, but as yet none have been found.

The problem facing scientists has been complicated by the fact that such chemicals produce cancers when mixed in a compound. In some cases, a carcinogenic agent such as hydrocarbon does not produce cancer by itself, but in combination with a certain oil, a material usually not cancer-producing, will promptly produce one. This precludes the possibility that the federal government can simply regulate or prohibit use of these chemicals. Recently, chemicals have been uncovered that prevent or retard the action of cancer-producing chemicals. The large amount of research and investigation required in this area eventually lead to the discovery of chemicals that will prevent the development of cancer in individuals who are unavoidably and sometimes unknowingly exposed to certain cancer-producing substances.

In addition to all of the work that will be necessary to help in the diagnosis and treatment of cancer today, there must be an unstinting loyalty to the basic research that is necessary to provide the long-term answers to cancer. But, for the consumers of today (1974), care must be the best we can provide. And the experts at the National Cancer Institute feel this requires physicians to take a team approach. We can no longer consider surgery or radiation — the well-known therapies of the past — to be effective singly in all cases. We must make surgery *and* radiation *and* chemotherapy available right from the start. In order to provide what the consumer will need in the short-term future (the next five to ten years) we must also turn to the chemist or chemotherapist, and the research being done in drug treatment. For the long term (beyond the next decade) we must go to the basic scientists, particularly the immunologists and the geneticists. To do any less than concentrating on all three time periods would be cheating ourselves.

Dr. Frank J. Rauscher, Jr., Director of the National Cancer Institute, provided vivid testimony on the effects of cutbacks in describing the impact of the administration's reduction of the 1974 budget for the national cancer program. Dr. Rauscher states that the reduction would "adversely affect the great momentum that has developed and the expectations of the staff, the scientific community, the Congress, and the informed public. . . . A reduced budget would restrict the clinical trials in immunologic treatment. Detection and treatment in immunology offer the most immediate promise for major cancers."

Research on immunology has produced some of the greatest triumphs of modern medicine. It has enabled physicians to protect people against a wide variety of bacteria and viruses. The field of immunology began with the observation that individuals who got a disease such as smallpox were safe from catching the disease again; they were immune. It may someday be possible to make people immune to cancer or to use their immune systems to cure their disease if they do get cancer.

Dr. Rauscher testified that: "Good to excellent results — as measured by early and long-term evaluations — are being obtained in the control of fifteen different cancers when four or five anti-cancer drugs are applied in combination, or when these drugs are used in addition to surgery, radiation therapy, or immunotherapy. We would have to delay (if the Nixon budget prevailed) the testing of new clinical anti-tumor agents in man."

59

The 1971 report of the National Panel of Consultants on the Conquest of Cancer indicated that new drugs and drug treatment comprise one of the areas of greatest importance in cancer research. Several human tumors have been cured by drugs alone, which led the Panel to conclude that there is a potential for cure by the use of drugs. Research on which drug to give for which tumor, in what combinations, and when in the course of the disease (for example, before an operation, after an operation, in combination with radiotherapy or not, etc.) it should be given, are areas of great importance.

Dr. Michael B. Shimkin, in his excellent book *The Cancer Story,* points out that it was not until 1955 that a large government-supported national program of cancer chemotherapy (drug treatment) was organized in the United States. He divides the drug treatment of cancer into four steps: selecting the chemicals or other materials to be tested; testing the material in animal tumors; determining the proper dosage and any side effects of agents showing anti-tumor effects in animals; and evaluating the use of drugs on cancer patients who no longer can be helped by established forms of treatment.

It becomes readily apparent from the above description of the steps by which a cancer drug is developed that it is not a short process. Therefore, to delay the testing of new anti-cancer drugs, as the Nixon Administration has proposed, means a very long delay in utilizing these drugs.

Dr. Rauscher stated that: "Evidence is rapidly accumulating that at least four newly-discovered candidate viruses may cause cancer in man. If this is true, it can lead to the development of methods for preventing specific types of cancer. These leads cannot be developed or studied, and attacks on new viruses which may induce human malignancies cannot be mounted at the $550 million level." (The actual Nixon Administration request was for even less, $500 million.)

We still lack proof that human cancer is caused by a virus, despite fruitful and continuing research in this area. If we are able to identify a virus responsible for any form of human cancer, it could open the door to the development of vaccines for its prevention. This is no longer a wild dream, but is well within the realistic possibilities of future research.

Rauscher further testified: "Recent developments in molecular biology have increased our understanding of the cancer process and have opened up new leads for the control of malignancy. Efforts to fully exploit these leads would be limited (by the budget cuts)."

Scientists tell us that a major goal of cancer research is to find specific and constant differences between normal and cancer cells, differences that are essential to the development and maintenance of malignancy. It seems that all living cells have been shown capable of becoming cancerous, and therefore basic research is of special importance to the understanding of this malignant disease which is characterized by uncontrolled growth. Somehow, normal cells know when to stop dividing. But cancer cells are unruly. They do not have an orderly behavior; they often grow in clumps and pile up on each other, forming big tumors. They may even choke off the food and oxygen supply that normal cells need, thereby killing them.

Laboratory scientists are trying to learn why cancer cells behave the way they do by transplanting cancers from one animal to another. Scientists are also looking into individual cells and have information about their different parts, including the nucleus with its DNA and RNA, and the mitochondria and ribosomes. These are currently very active areas of basic research.

Other important areas include research on hormones and on cellular nutrition. Nutrition studies, for example, have shown that one amino acid is manufactured by normal cells but is not manufactured by cancer cells. This research has led to some important advances in dealing with patients with acute leukemia.

Dr. Michael DeBakey summed up the importance of medical research as follows:

Our ultimate goal is not treatment but prevention; we want to eliminate the factors which cause heart disease, stroke, cancer, and the numerous other fatal or disabling diseases. America has an abundance of fine minds eager to study these conditions. Scientists and technicians must be trained to do research. This investment is one of the wisest we can make, for our failure to invest in finding the causes and cures of disease increases our expenditures for patient care without increasing our effectiveness. Ultimately, you (the consumer) are the beneficiary; the new knowledge uncovered in the research laboratory will eventually be used to clinical advantage.

The National Cancer Act of 1971 is a logical step in accelerating the government's attack on cancer. In the thirty-four intervening years from the establishment of NCI to the passage of this Cancer Conquest Act, the population of the United States has more than doubled. In 1935, the cancer death toll was estimated to be 153,000 people, and for 1969, it was estimated to be 323,000. In 1936, the cancer death toll in my home city of Seattle was estimated at 710, and in 1969, it was 1,350 for Seattle, and over 5,000 for the residents of the State of Washington.

These statistics do not indicate a great deal of progress over the years. Figures are often deceptive, especially in areas like this, where even today accurate statistics are difficult to secure.

The situation in research is now far different from that in 1937. The Congress established the Cancer Institute in what was almost a scientific research vacuum. Medical research was almost non-existent. Today, the Cancer Institute is an integral part of the National Institutes of Health (NIH), where we conduct and support research into the whole spectrum of diseases that plague mankind: heart, lung, arthritis, infectious diseases, neurological, kidney, eye — all of these individual, yet interrelated, illnesses are studied and researched in the most professional manner possible by the most competent people available.

If anyone needs further affirmation or reaffirmation of the need for a national program for the conquest of cancer, the final report of the National Panel of Consultants published in 1971 should serve the purpose. The summary indicated:

Cancer is the number one health concern of the American people. Of the 200 million Americans alive today, 50 million will develop cancer at present rates of incidence, and 34 million will die of this painful and often ugly disease if better methods of prevention and treatment are not discovered. About one-half of cancer deaths occur before the age of 65, and cancer causes more deaths among children under age 15 than any other illness. Over 16 percent of all deaths in the United States are caused by cancer. Cancer often strikes as harshly at human dignity as at human life, and more often than not, it represents financial catastrophe for the family in which it strikes.

In terms of setting national priorities, the panel report had this to say:

The amount spent on cancer research is grossly inadequate today. For every man, woman and child in the United States, we spent in 1969: $410 on national defense, $19 on the space program, $19 on foreign aid, and $.89 on cancer research. Cancer deaths last year (1971) were eight times the number of lives lost in six years in Viet Nam, five-and-one-half times the number killed in automobile accidents, and greater than the number of Americans killed in battle in all four years of World War II. Given the seriousness of the cancer problem to the health and morale of our society, this allocation of national priorities seems open to serious question.

This special thrust in cancer should not be at the expense of research into other important medical areas. It should also be clearly stated that this cancer conquest should not be at the expense of programs such as the regional medical program designed to bring the latest in medical technology to the population at large.

I advocate the highest position for research as part of our comprehensive health policy. This would make it clear that America intends to retain its pre-eminence in medical research, and will be the nation most responsible for eliminating what Senator Neely called the "most terrifying scourge that has ever threatened the existence of the human race."

Many experts believe that, with full application of our known methods of diagnosing and treating cancer, we would be able today to save 50 percent of all cancer patients. This possibility demands the development of better methods of public health education and medical care. These goals, and the study of ways in which to achieve them, are as important as is the research on the cell. But saving 50 percent, although good for 1974, should not be good enough for 1985. We need to aim for 100 percent.

The letter which I received from Dr. William J. Mayo (founder of the Mayo Clinic) when I first introduced the creation of the National Cancer Institute still holds today:

> My brother, Dr. Charles H. Mayo, and I, and our associates in the clinic are very glad that you have introduced this bill, *the purpose of which is of the greatest importance to the welfare of the people of this country and to the world.* Too much cannot be said in favor of proper means and measures to learn the cause of cancer and to cure and prevent the disease.

5.   The Environment

Washington Post, March 21, 1972: "Viruses Peril Water of Two Massachusetts Cities."

Louisville Courier-Journal and Times, December 17, 1972: "State's Drinking Water Program Brought 'F' From EPA Last May."

Atlanta Constitution, January 3, 1973: "After Schools Epidemic, Water Hepatitis Test Sought."

San Mateo Times, January 3, 1973: "How Pure Is Our Water?"

These headlines emerged from hearings before the U.S. Senate Commerce Committee on my bill, entitled the "Safe Drinking Water Act of 1973."

The Senate Commerce Committee, and particularly its Subcommittee on the Environment, has become increasingly occupied with pursuing and conserving our natural resources. These activities are geared to meet the goals declared in the National Environmental Policy Act of 1969. In that Act, Congress declared that we will encourage productive and enjoyable harmony between man and his environment, to promote efforts which will prevent or eliminate damage to the environment and stimulate the health and welfare of man.

Ruth C. Cluson, Chairman of the Environmental Quality Committee of the League of Women Voters of the United States, presented the following statement to our Committee during the hearings on safe drinking water, which would seem to represent the feelings of all people in this country:

> Members of the League of Women Voters of the United States, along with most Americans, accept tap water anywhere in this country to be safe and palatable. Because we have been studying water quality for years, we know that the facts do not corroborate these expectations.

We now know that water supplies can become polluted in many ways; that quality standards differ throughout the country; and that citizens for the most part simply do not know whether or not their drinking water meets any standards.

In March 1973, two severe community problems traceable to unsafe drinking water occurred in Florida. In one, 97 cases of typhoid were reported in a migrant labor camp twenty-five miles south of Miami. The other was the discovery of high bacterial counts in Miami Beach drinking water, with the warning to drink only boiled water.

From 1961 to 1970, there were 128 known outbreaks of disease or poisoning traceable to drinking water. Twenty people died, and an estimated 46,374 became ill. It is safe to assume that many additional cases were not even reported.

In 1969, a U.S. Public Health Service study disclosed that over half (56%) of 969 public waterworks surveyed had physical deficiencies; over half (51%) failed to disinfect their water; and one-sixth (15%) exceeded one or more mandatory limits in federal drinking water standards.

The study continues:

> . . . Most deficiencies were found in smaller waterworks which often lack staff, equipment and funds to improve their operation. Of the 40,000 waterworks in the nation, 1,300 large systems serve 106 million people, while the rest supply only 54 million people. This leaves 50 million people dependent on individual home supplies. An estimated 20 million Americans have inadequate plumbing facilities.

The General Accounting Office (GAO) has been studying safe drinking water for the past two years. Although my own state was not the only one to come within the scope of their investigation. I do want to comment briefly on their findings in Washington State.

(1) Of the 127 systems surveyed, only seven could pass Washington State bacteriological standards.

(2) 65 percent of Washington's systems had not had a chemical analysis — mercury, cadmium, lead, organic chemicals, etc. — performed within the past year. Existing standards call for analyses at least once a year.

(3) The State does not require that sanitary surveys be made of treatment plants. It relies solely on reports given to the State by the water supply systems themselves, and then only from the larger systems.

(4) Although 400 of Washington's larger water supply systems have been instructed by the State to establish programs to prevent contamination through unforeseen reductions in pressure, only three of the systems had effective programs as of October 1972.

(5) Only four percent of Washington State's water supply system operators were certified as of July 1972. While the state standards do not address themselves to this issue, responsible thinking indicates that virtually all operators responsible for water treatment plants should be certified.

Virtually the same conclusions were found in the other states as well. GAO looked at bottled drinking water and drinking water supplied at federal facilities. Both were found lacking.

Many of the problems cited in the GAO Report could be solved under the Program Grants section of my Safe Drinking Water proposal. Money would be available to the states to finance up to two-thirds of their drinking water program costs.

Henry Eschwege, Director of the Resources and Economics Division of the GAO, presented the following evaluation of the legislation:

67

We believe that the legislation before this Subcommitee is designed to provide reasonable solutions to the problems that our investigation has identified. The legislation would require the establishment of national drinking water standards designed to reasonably protect the public health; and national secondary standards designed to reasonably assure aesthetically adequate drinking water. The legislation provides that states have primary responsibility for enforcing the standards, but it authorizes the federal government to enforce the primary standards if the state fails to take corrective action after receiving notice that a public drinking water system does not comply with the primary standard.

It is important to point out that this legislation in no way intends to infringe upon the state's rights and local responsibilities in this area. It is meant to establish the standards that provide minimum public health and safety safeguards to the public.

The community water supply study of 1969 first brought to our attention the potentially detrimental effects of chronic exposure to trace contaminants which are normally not removed by existing water treatment methods under the best of conditions. The study indicated that viruses and toxic organic compounds have been repeatedly found in drinking water even after what is called "complete treatment."

Ralph Nader focused on this point in testifying before our Committee:

It is not difficult to appreciate why these recalcitrant contaminants escape the purification process. Current technology relies almost exclusively upon innovations of the latter 19th and early 20th centuries, when treatment focused on the need to remove bacterial pathogens.

Although half of the population in the United States receives its drinking water from surface water supplies, most of these are contaminated by organic wastes and little is known about the effect of ingesting these organics for long periods of time.

One of the few studies on the physiological effects of organic fractions in treated drinking water was conducted by W.C. Huper and W.W. Payne on the water supply of Nitro, W. Va., so named because there is a Du Pont plant there, on the Kanawha River. By demonstrating the cancer-causing, life-shortening properties of these organic fractions, they suggested:

> Comprehensive studies for obtaining valid information must be undertaken in order to forestall a possible future development of a potentially catastrophic cancer epidemic among the general population of communities or regions exposed to carcinogens (cancer-causing agents) from such sources.

J.B. Andelman and M.J. Suess, writing in the Bulletin of the World Health Organization (WHO), sounded a similar alarm:

> When one considers that animal experiments have shown that repeated exposure to carcinogens is more effective than an equivalent single dose, one should not neglect the possibility of cancer from the repeated lifelong exposure to carcinogens in air, food, and water.

In examining potential disease-causing substances in drinking water, Ralph Nader stated:

> I consider drinking water contamination one of the top five consumer issues in the United States . . . Sampling from the tap water at the United States Public Health Service Hospital at Carville and at the Carrolltown Purification Plant in New Orleans, the Environmental Protection Agency identified as many as forty synthetic organic compounds in the drinking water.
>
> Six of these compounds have been shown to produce pathological (disease-causing) changes in animals in chronic toxicity (poisons) studies, and three of these compounds have been shown to be carcinogenic (cancer-causing).
>
> Perhaps it is not surprising that New Orleans has

been reported to rank third highest of 163 metropolitan areas for incidence of kidney cancer, sixth highest for cancer of the bladder and urinary organs, ninth highest for cancer of unspecified digestive organs, and has 2.6 times the national average incidence of tongue cancer fatalities, and 3.5 times the national average incidence of cancer of other parts of the mouth.

None of these reports sums up the hard-to-calculate costs of impaired health, lost days of work, and reduced standard of living traceable to substandard water supply. Protecting the public requires that we also consider these factors.

Existing technology is capable of substantial removal of toxic organics and viruses. The question might well be raised, then, why this technology is not being used.

Ralph Nader observes a seemingly widespread attitude in the waterworks fraternity that "what you can't see won't hurt you." Others operate on the philosophy that a contaminant must be proven harmful before action is required. Somehow, they are able to reconcile themselves to the fact that the public becomes the "guinea pig" in this environmental version of Russian roulette.

I think it is important to draw upon the exciting recent work being done at the National Cancer Institute, where research has shown possible connections between viruses and cancer. The question often arises as to where the viruses come from: maybe they come from water, and maybe they build up over time. We must be diligent in seeking the ways a virus can get into the human body, and drinking water, if not properly treated, must be a prime suspect.

More public information is needed about our resources, including the drinking water supply. There seems to be an operating assumption that you don't want to tell the public about bad conditions because it will unduly alarm them. But this is not the correct approach. It is far better to keep the public informed so that they will support elected and appointed officials in their efforts to improve water quality.

The Seattle Water Department, for example, makes an

annual report to the City Council. Generally no hearing is held on whether anything has been done to upgrade water quality. Public awareness should require that when water treatment systems present their reports, they should also be quizzed on improvements which have been and should be made. If, in the future, a bond issue is voted to upgrade the system, the public will be aware and certainly more receptive if they know the facts.

The problems of our health and the environment are just beginning to be examined in a comprehensive fashion by the federal government. It is important to treat this discussion of safe drinking water as an example of many other areas of the environment which need new public health and safety protections.

The Senate Commerce Committee is looking into several subjects in depth. We are now taking the attitude that air, water, soil and our natural surroundings can no longer be taken for granted. The public must be protected from hazards in their environment, particularly those which man is creating himself. It is pleasing for me to note that the Safe Drinking Water Act, which I introduced along with twenty-one cosponsors, passed the Senate in June of 1973. I look forward to these provisions becoming the law of the land. The proposal applies federal minimum standards to all public drinking water supplies, and calls for the individual states to be primarily responsible for their enforcement. The federal government would only step in if states fail to see that drinking water supplies are in fact safe.

Robert Sherrill, writing for the *New York Times* in January 1973, described a New York tire company executive fictitiously named Charles Armin. Armin, who had never been seriously ill in his life, was a 200-pound robust and healthy fellow who looked much younger than his 60 years. He enjoyed sailing in his spare time, and ran a taut ship on the job, too. He first went to see a doctor in December 1971 because of sharp pains in his chest. The tests showed his heart in fine shape and the lung x-rays showed nothing wrong. The pains

71

grew worse. In April 1972, doctors found Mr. Armin suffering from mesothelioma, a cancer so rare that it is not listed separately in the medical classifications. It is a cancer of the chest lining or of the stomach lining. People with it will die within a year because it either covers the entire lung area or infuses the whole abdomen. Mr. Armin was dead 14 weeks after mesothelioma was discovered. Health experts have now been able to uncover the cause. It was asbestos.

Asbestos has not been seen as a villain by most Americans. It has served to fire-proof clothing and insulation in buildings, and to make brake linings on automobiles safer and more durable. But it is now becoming clear that asbestos has a sinister side. It can serve as a catalyst to lung cancer, to asbestosis, and to mesothelioma, the disease described above. It has also been found that asbestos exaggerates the cancer-causing effects of tobacco smoke to make it much more difficult for someone in contact with both asbestos and cigarette smoke to escape getting cancer.

There are 5,000,000 Americans whose jobs require that they breathe a significant amount of asbestos dust. These include construction workers, oil refinery workers, and insulation workers. One disturbing aspect of Mr. Armin's story is how he first became exposed to asbestos. During World War II, he served as a tinsmith in the Brooklyn Navy Yard, helping to install fiberglass in destroyers' refrigeration holds. There are over 3,000,000 other Americans who worked in shipyards during World War II, and some scientists feel that we may be on the way toward a large number of similar cases. Dr. Irving Selikoff, a professor at Mt. Sinai School of Medicine in New York, one of the leading experts in this field, points out that in Great Britain, there are a large number of mesothelioma patients. These currently number over 1,600. The ominous cloud here is that residents in Great Britain began working in shipyards about 1935, almost five years earlier than in the United States.

Asbestos dust can be sucked up through hoods over machines in factories and captured in bags. This bagging can be done without human hands getting involved in this process.

The federal government has instituted standards for factories to keep the asbestos fibre count below five fibres per cubic centimeter. Many experts are now questioning whether five fibres is not too high, and some have even advocated that this standard be lowerd to two fibres.

Dr. Selikoff appeared before our Senate Commerce Committee in February 1973 to testify on behalf of my Toxic Substances Control Act. At that time. Dr. Selikoff described the multiplier effect:

> Asbestos workers are at risk to cancer of the abdomen and cancer of the chest due to the cancer effects of the asbestos. Yet, if they don't smoke cigarettes, they don't die of cancer of the lungs, or at least not very much. On the other hand, if they also smoke cigarettes, they die of cancer of the lung about eight times as often as all other cigarette smokers. We have found that asbestos workers who smoke cigaretts have about 92 times the risk of dying of lung cancer compared to people who neither smoke cigarettes nor work with asbestos.
>
> In the last five years in this country, studying all the insulation workers, we have found that one out of every five deaths among them is due to lung cancer. Indeed, if you add the other cancers, almost one out of every two insulation workers in this country who has died in the last five years has died of cancer. This is a disaster.

The Toxic Substances Control Act is designed to restrict the distribution of poisonous chemicals and to screen manufacturers' safety data prior to the production of new chemicals. This would allow the prevention of hazards before they become manifest. Asbestos is only one of several chemicals that need to be looked at closely. Phosphates in detergents are largely responsible for the premature aging of lakes. Mercury in consumer products is responsible for a large amount of the mercury pollution now present in our lakes and streams. Other problem chemicals include polychlorinated bithenyls, a family of compounds that in many ways resemble DDT. They have contaminated hundreds of thousands of chickens. The common characteristic of all of these chemical compounds is that there is currently no adequate authority to control their manufacture, use, and disposal.

A problem such as asbestos dust was in the past of little interest to anyone except the worker himself. But, if we are going to do the best that we can for the health of our nation, then we must attack the illnesses that beset us because of air and water pollution, pesticides, land degradation, and hazards of the workplace.

Congress, recognizing the importance of the workplace, passed the Occupational Safety and Health Act in 1970. This Act declared that it was the intent of Congress to "assure, so far as possible, to every working man and woman in the nation safe and healthful working conditions, and to preserve our human resources."

Chemicals such as mercury and asbestos require that we look not only at the workplace or at chemicals in the air or water, but also at the total risk of exposure from such substances. That is why we need a special focus on toxic substances.

Asbestos dust is a good example of a useful substance which can cause horrible suffering and death under certain circumstances. Its usefulness is great, but that is no excuse for failing to take action to protect people against the health hazards it creates.

The automobile is another example of a mixed blessing. Automobiles are, obviously, important to the American economy and the quality of American life. One has only to look at the turmoil caused by recent gasoline shortages to realize how central to living the automobile is in America today. But the automobile is also a killer. It is the number one cause of accidental death among people between the ages of 15 and 44, and it is a major killer of people of all ages (27 percent of persons aged 0-4; 49 percent of those aged 6-14; 72 percent of those aged 15-24; 57 percent of those aged 25-44; and 46 percent of those aged 45-65). For every person who is killed in a car accident, there are several who are so severely injured that they will not work or play, happily and without pain, for the rest of their days. The death and disability, the suffering and loss of income and enjoyment caused by motor vehicles, is enormous and unnecessary. We can and must take further steps to increase the safety of motor vehicle travel in the United States. We must create for ourselves, for the 2,000,000 Americans who are involved in motor vehicle accidents each year, an emergency health services system at least as good as the one the U.S. operated for wounded GI's in Vietnam. Thousands of auto accident victims are dying each year of "recoverable injuries" because of deficiencies in the quality and delivery of emergency health services. A recent study found that no rehabilitiation program at all was suggested to 88.6 percent of seriously injured motor vehicle accident victims. We must create adequate rehabilitation services for the victims of motor vehicle accidents, so that they can be restored to a useful and productive life.

In 1972, there were 56,000 fatalities from motor vehicle accidents. The total cost, including human suffering and grief to the survivors of the deceased, is incalculable. The strictly financial loss, for one year's highway carnage, is estimated at $17.5 billion. That includes estimated wage losses, medical expenses, administrative and settlement costs, and property damage.

We are convinced that automobiles can and must be manufactured more safely. We are also convinced that we need a completely new system of treatment and compensation for the victims of traffic accidents, one that would save and restore lives and move quickly to replace the lost pay checks of the hospitalized motorist.

That new system is "no-fault" automobile insurance, although it might better be called "no-lawsuit" automobile insurance because it is your own insurance company that must pay you for your personal injury losses without a lawsuit to prove who was at fault. Instead of the complicated (and expensive) process of establishing negligence and freedom from contributory negligence and payment from liability insurance, we would go back to the oldest and best known form of insurance — one in which you buy insurance against loss to yourself and those close to you. Life insurance, fire insurance, theft insurance, and health insurance are all forms of "no-fault" insurance, and this should be the case for motor vehicle insurance. Today the American people spend $1.5 billion a year on lawyers' fees to fight over who was at fault in automobile accidents. A no-fault auto insurance system would turn that money into emergency health services and rehabilitation facilities for victims and into premium reductions for motorists.

The President of the American College of Emergency Physicians, Dr. James Mills, testified before the Senate Commerce Committee in 1973 that a nationwide no-fault auto insurance system would, by timely payment of all medical costs to victims, greatly improve the adequacy of emergency medical care. National no-fault should necessarily follow the law which Congress passed that same year providing grants to develop better methods of emergency care and training programs for emergency health personnel. Health professionals cannot be expected to wait twelve months or more to be paid (the average time it takes to settle an automobile negligence claim) and payment should not depend on whether the victim is found by a jury to have been "free from contributory negligence." The person who buys an auto insurance policy has the right to expect that his insurance company will pay for all the emergency facilities and equipment and personnel that it takes to save his life, and for all the communications equipment, mobile medical facilities, and modern transport that it takes to get his child into surgery quickly to assure full recovery, rather than condemnation to a lifetime as a cripple.

Under my plan to establish national no-fault motor vehicle insurance, every victim of an automobile accident anywhere in the United States will have the financial resources to pay for the best emergency transportation and medical services available. At the same time, every private hospital and ambulance service will be assured of timely payment on behalf of every such victim rather than only from those who are rich or who are eventually found eligible for compensation under today's outmoded liability insurance system. A recent study in the State of Vermont found that "twenty-three percent (of highway victims) died of probably survivable injuries due to problems through the emergency care system" and that "almost half" of those who were taken from the scene of the accident alive but who died afterward "died of injuries that were either definitely or possibly survivable."

Just think what it could mean if, through a modern form of no-lawsuit compensation, we could save the lives of 23 percent of the highway victims who are "scheduled" to die in 1975 or 1976 or 1977. One of those lives could be yours — or that of a loved one.

The President of the Appalachian Regional Hospitals, Theodore P. Hipkins, testified before the Senate Commerce Committee that:

> ...the principal advantage of a no-fault system of automobile insurance is that all parties involved in the system — the accident victim, the insurer, the state and agencies providing help and rehabilitative service — have positive incentives to restore the individual who is involved in an accident to maximum physical and occupational functions as rapidly as possible.

Compare that with the U.S. Department of Transportation's finding about the negligence-liability insurance system:

> The traditional (system) offers nothing to encourage and much to preclude the early introduction of rehabilitation ... considerable time, energy, and expense must be devoted to controversy just when rehabilitation measures might most benefit the victim.

It is sad to contemplate, but there are cases where auto accident victims short-sightedly fail to start rehabilitation programs because, if they recover and are, for example, able to walk again, the jury might not award them as big a damage verdict. In all too many cases these misguided victims never will walk again because it is probably too late for rehabilita-

77

tion if they wait until the jury returns its verdict. A proper medical and rehabilitation services program must be started almost immediately and adhered to faithfully if it is to succeed. The biggest irony of all is that as much as one-half of that big damage verdict won't go to the victim — but to his lawyer.

It may well be that the single most significant contribution of nationwide no-fault insurance, once it becomes law, will be the improved availability and adequacy of rehabilitation services for victims.

Under my proposal, for the first time, every victim of an automobile accident will be able to afford and will be encouraged by both his own insurance company and the State agency in charge of vocational rehabilitation to use and take advantage of a complete range of medical and vocational rehabilitation services. Prompt referral, an accountability program, and incentives to victims to return to work all should be combined to reduce the tragic human waste that occurs when victims remain totally or partially disabled rather than resuming rewarding and productive lives.

Dr. Justus F. Lehmann, the Chairman of the Department of Rehabilitation Medicine at the University of Washington, wrote me that he and his colleagues were strongly in favor of no-fault insurance because:

we see the terrible aftermath of automobile accidents which may ruin not only the life of an individual but also the future of entire families.

This bill can drastically change the dismal picture which is presented by these patients. The real problem is that the cost of getting these people back on their feet to work or to school is formidable. They end up on welfare . . . in many instances whole families are forced on the welfare payroll.

The President of the Blue Cross Association of America, Walter J. McNerney, testified before the Senate Commerce Committee that no-fault insurance:

will encourage quality of care, will give the consumer his

choice, and **will** assist the public to get its money's worth out of every health care dollar.

It is also a way to cut down on the mental anguish and strain experienced by everyone who has been in an automobile accident. The victim will not have to worry about how his family is going to be able to meet the mortgage payments and buy food while he is convalescing. Freeing the victim from such economic anxieties means he can concentrate all his energies on getting well, and he will in fact recover more quickly and completely.

Surprisingly, in view of all these benefits, if the nation shifts to no-fault, the average motorist in every one of the fifty states will pay a lower annual insurance premium. An independent firm of actuaries, Milliman and Robertson, Inc., was retained by the U.S. Department of Transportation to prepare a cost estimate of my no-fault insurance bill. In every state, adoption of the federal standards set forth would mean a premium reduction. Under my proposal, all reasonable medical and rehabilitation services, wage loss compensation up to $15,000, reasonable amounts for replacement services, and a reasonable amount for death benefits would be assured.

If we are going to look at preventive medicine and public health in their broadest aspects, then we must identify the necessary social and environmental factors that will promote good health. It is in this context that a program such as no-fault insurance should be seen to determine its beneficial impact on health and costs of health to consumers. A significant impact upon such mass killers as lung cancer, emphysema, heart disease and automobile accidents depends on modifications of environmental factors as well as long-term medical cures. Examples are legion. An innovation such as the impact-absorbing steering column on an automobile may well reduce the number of deaths from accidents by the thousands and the number of crippling injuries by hundreds of thousands. The use of a simple safety closure for aspirin, soaps, detergents and cleaners, vitamins and irons, bleaches and insecticides, has been shown to reduce child poisoning by as much as 86 percent. Industrial accidents in this country claim 39 lives each day; a substantial number are victims of needlessly unsafe working conditions. Again, elimination of deadly salmonella, an objective well within our technical capacity, would substantially reduce the incidence of serious food poisoning in the United States.

As Chairman of the Health, Education and Welfare Appropriations Subcommittee, I have had the opportunity to examine and study the preventive health services supplied through the federal Public Health Service. These programs are housed within the Center for Disease Control (CDC), which includes the National Institute of Occupational Safety and Health, and the Community Environmental Management Agency. The CDC over the past quarter century has compiled a superior record of accomplishments in the national effort to prevent disease and to protect the health of the public. It is unfortunate that, during budget year 1974, the Administration proposed to reduce the budget of this agency by $4 million. Congress restored a large portion of this in order to allow the CDC to investigate viral and bacterial diseases and support activities in the immunization field.

A new and important part of CDC is the National Institute of Occupational Safety and Health (NIOSH). This agency is developing criteria for safety and health standards for the workplace, stimulating professional manpower development and evaluating hazards to individual workers, industries, and unions. As our society becomes more and more complex, the need for consumers to have greater protection increases substantially. The examples described in this chapter indicate how much farther government has to go before we can insure a more healthy environment for our citizens.

6.   Consumer Safety and Protection

> Consumers are the only important group in the economy who are not effectively organized, whose views are often not heard . . . Additional legislative and administrative action is required if the federal government is to meet its responsibility to consumers in the exercise of their rights. These rights include: the right to safety — the right to be informed — the right to choose — the right to be heard.
>
> President John F. Kennedy, Consumer
> Message to Congress, March 15, 1962

The National Commission on Product Safety was appointed by President Lyndon B. Johnson on March 27, 1968 under legislation that I introduced. In establishing this Commission, Congress recognized that modern technology poses a threat to the physical security of consumers. In filing their report two years later, the Commission found:

> The threat of technology to the consumer is bona fide and menacing. Moreover, we believe that, without effective governmental intervention, the abundance and variety of unreasonable hazards associated with consumer products cannot be reduced to a level befitting a just and civilized society.

The main concern of the Commission was to set up a unit in government that would protect the consumer from product hazards, focusing on household hazards and hazardous household products. This area is the third leg of the tripod of major causes of accidents, the other two being vehicular products, especially the automobile, and accidents relating to the workplace.

The Commission found:

Americans — 20 million of them — are injured each year in the home as a result of incidents connected with consumer products. Of the total, 110,000 are permanently disabled, and 30,000 are killed. A significant number could have been spared if more attention had been paid to hazard reduction. The annual cost to the nation of product-related injuries may exceed $5.5 billion. The exposure of consumers to unreasonable consumer product hazards is excessive by any standard of measurement."

The National Commission on Product Safety attempted to discover how household hazards could be identified. For example, they looked into home fires and found that annually 6,200 people were killed and 1,300,000 injured by burns received at home. What were the causes: matches, stoves, wiring, fabric, cigarettes?

Falls at home accounted for approximately 12,000 deaths and injuries to almost 7 million people. But again, what were the causes? High-heels, loose threads, rough floors, flimsy ladders, worn stairs, slippery floors, torn carpet, alcohol?

The most dangerous years are below the age of five. Approximately 7,000 children die each year in home accidents, a death toll that is higher than the child mortality rate for cancer and heart disease combined. More than two million children each year are injured by bicycles or playground equipment.

About one-third of the deaths from household hazards occur in kitchens and living/dining areas. Stairs account for about one in every twenty deaths from household hazards, and slightly fewer deaths occur in the bathroom. Falls figure in half of these deaths, fires or suffocation in one-third, poisoning in about one in twenty.

These hard statistics convey no sense of the agony and suffering of the victims and their families. The Commission went out of its way to indicate how deeply moved its members were by accounts of individual lives destroyed or blighted by defective household products.

Consumer safety, of course, is a valid subject for any book about the public's health, because it is a form of preventive medicine. A doctor friend once observed to me that one good piece of consumer protection legislation could save more lives than a hundred physicians — and, with full appreciation for the good works of American doctors, I believe he was right.

Let us look at some areas that affect children.

At the first hearing of the Commission in New York City, Dr. Allan B. Coleman, Chairman of the American Academy of Pediatrics' Committee on Accident Prevention, voiced alarm over hazards associated with new bicycle design. Among other observations, he stated:

> The currently popular bicycles with high-rise handlebars are causing undue numbers of cheek injuries.

A few months earlier, Dr. T.R. Howell had reported an "epidemic" of injuries to the skull and face among children using bicycles with small front wheels, low-set front axles, long narrow seats, and high, wide handlebars. The American Academy of Pediatrics at that time asked that a "hard look" be taken at the design of some of these new bicycles. The Public Health Service estimates that bicycles are associated with approximately 1 million injuries each year, including 120,000 fractures and 60,000 concussions. The Physicians Survey put bicycles first on the list of products associated with injuries treated by doctors in their offices.

Testimony before the Commission brought out case after case where household chemicals found their way with disaster into little children's mouths.

83

Clancy Emert, a one year old toddler in Peoria, Illinois, swallowed about three tablespoons of Old English furniture and scratch-cover polish in a moment when his aunt left the bottle unguarded. The petroleum distillates collected in his lungs. He died 40 hours later of chemical pneumonia.

One year old Peter Schwab of Seattle, Washington, dipped his finger into the soap dispenser of an automatic dishwasher and tasted the undischarged electrasol detergent. His mother, a few feet away, heard him scream and quickly flushed his mouth at the tap. Peter spent two days in Children's Orthopedic Hospital's intensive care units for treatment for alkaline burns and blisters of his mouth. His parent's quick action possibly saved his life.

Because young children are so curious, household chemicals pose a major hazard. Every liquid or chewable substance is something for them to sample.

I would never want anyone else to be put through the pain and grief which we had and still always will have. It was a horrible nightmare.

This letter from a mother whose infant son was strangled by the top of his own crib unfortunately was not unique.

Nationwide, as many as 200 deaths each year may be laid to crib strangulation. In Dade County, Florida alone, crib slats, sides or tops have strangled at least one infant each year for the past ten years.

Even when a parent of a victim acts to correct the danger of design, he may be ignored. A father whose son was killed within three weeks of the incident described above in the same fashion and by the same model crib told the Commission:

After the death of our son we tried for several months to get a voluntary commitment to make this product safe or not to make it (at all) out of the manufacturer. We tried the pressure of a law suit and a financial settlement was made; but our primary concern about the safety of the product went unsatisfied.

The National Commission identified the cirb that was involved in both tragedies. It was Pride-Trimble's Kiddy Koop, a nationally distributed product. Ironically, its motto displayed prominently on the front page of its catalog is: "Since 1912, your baby's health and comfort our only business."

According to the Commission's in-depth study of 215 injuries reported from infant furniture — which includes high chairs, walkers, cribs, playpens and dressing tables — 84 percent of the victims were less than five years old. Almost 60 percent incurred injuries to the head or face; more than half of all injuries were head lacerations or contusions and abrasions. The product was adjudged at fault by the Commission staff in two-thirds of the injuries investigated.

A study conducted by Dr. Harvey Kravitz at Northwestern University Medical School found that more than 1,750,000 infants, or just under half of all current births, will annually sustain at least one bad fall during the first year of life. Ill-designed high chairs, play chairs or dressing tables increase an infant's chances for such a fall. Skull fracture, nerve damage and permanent brain injury have been observed. Kravitz found that manufacturers appear to design infant furniture with insufficient regard to safety and primarily to impress the consumer with other attractions:

> The most common preventable accident was climbing out of a crib with the sides up. It would be unfair to consider these accidents as caused by human error. Much more attention should be given to designing cribs, taking into consideration the growth and development of infants. The "boxes with bars" of today have only four to six inch ratchets, the metal slides allowing height adjustment of the crib size. Longer ratchets should be added so that the mattress can be lowered closer to the floor and the sides raised higher.

Manufacturers of infant furniture should seriously

consider adding sides to the dressing table. The table might also have a concave surface instead of the present flat surface. Lowering the height is needed.

Few buyers are aware of the intrinsic hazards associated with infant's furniture. A witness before the Commission whose son was killed in a defective crib explained:

> A young couple going in to buy things for their first child is stepping into a world that is largely strange. They understand price and attractiveness; beyond that, very little. And yet, the decisions that they make can mean life or death for their child.
>
> Yet, in theory, we should have had a better than average chance to spot the danger. Both of us were older than the average age for a first child by quite a bit. Both of us had better than average education, and I have a mechanical ability sufficient enough that I earned my living while in college doing mechanical or repair work. Still, we did not realize the danger.

Parents reasonably assume that the juvenile furniture industry conducts tests and studies to determine effective design that will protect the child and still be attractive and economical. Instead, they are not even alerted to the risks of inadequate designs.

The U.S. Public Health Service estimates that toys injure 700,000 children every year; another 500,000 a year are injured on swings, and 200,000 on slides.

An attorney from Minneapolis alerted the Commission to the fact that at least twenty two parents are suing the manufacturer of an Etch-a-Sketch toy for lacerations suffered by their children from broken glass panels. In Philadelphia alone, at least thirteen children put the wrong end of a Zulu gun into their mouths and inhaled darts into their lungs. A Little Lady toy oven for young girls had temperatures above 300° Fahrenheit on the outer surface, and 600° Fahrenheit on the inside. There are no voluntary industry-wide safety standards for any of these products.

Hazards such as these led our Commerce Committe to enact the Child Protection and Toy Safety Act of 1969. This amended the federal Hazardous Substances Act to cover electrical, mechanical and thermal hazards from toys or other articles for children.

Injuries from toys often result from predictable misuse. It is safe to assume that a child would be expected to put the wrong end of a blow-gun into his mouth or to dismember a doll to expose sharp pins that hold the arms and legs.

In many ways, Charles W. Veysey, President of F.A.O. Schwartz Toy Store, spoke for most consumers when he stated:

> We can't take every toy and break it apart. We carry 12,000 different items. There are between 150,000 and 200,000 toys on the market to choose from. We have to rely on the manufacturer's integrity.

In formulating its recommendations, the Commission followed certain basic guidelines, namely:

—consumers have a right to safe products. When a manufacturer offers a product, the offer implies a warranty that the item is not unreasonably hazardous.

—protection against unreasonably hazardous consumer products should begin at the design stage before they are on the market.

—in assessing unreasonable hazards, the slight injury or the near miss may be as important as a calamity. It is not necessary to wait for an epidemic of injuries as proof of a hazard: expert technical judgment can often predict the risk.

—product safety is a joint enterprise of public agencies and the consumer; none acting alone can control unreasonable hazards.

—the government role in product safety is first to motivate businessmen to reduce product hazards while assuring fair treatment of competing interests; second, it is to promulgate and enforce safety regulations where voluntary efforts fail. At all times, the government should acquire, analyze, and release significant product safety information.

—the forces of competition and the profit motive are neither inherently conducive nor inimical to consumer protection. With government support, these forces can be channeled to assure compliance with safety standards to reduce unreasonable hazards.

—the public is entitled to predominant voice in decisions affecting its safety, specifically in the development of product safety standards.

—development of safety standards and regulation of product hazards serve all interests best if proceedings are open and on record, highly visible to everyone concerned.

-investments in product safety will yield a generous return on the capital required, possibly in an expanded market for consumer products, and certainly in the preservation of health and life.

With these underlying principles and guidelines in mind, the Commission recommended the establishment of an independent Consumer Product Safety Commission, and that the government be committed to eliminate unreasonable hazards found in and around the American home.

It was recommended that this new Commission be invested with authority to develop and set mandatory consumer product safety standards where industry's own efforts are not sufficient to protect consumers from unreasonable risks of death or injury.

Also recommended was an Injury Information Clearinghouse within the Consumer Product Safety Commission, with responsibility to collect and analyze data on product injuries, and to assure widespread distribution of information about defective products, the degree of hazards, and the nature of proposed remedies.

Following the receipt of this excellent report, I found that there was a very sound case for strong, innovative product safety legislation. The following week, Senator Frank E. Moss (D.-Utah), Chairman of the Commerce Consumer Subcommittee, and I introduced a bill encompassing the major suggestions of this report. Our measure also provided for the appointment of an independent "safety advocate" to represent consumer interests before the proposed Commission.

The Senate Commerce Committee began hearings on the bill in July 1971. It took a great deal of time to determine the powers that this new agency would have, and how it would relate and encompass a good deal of prior legislation in these areas.

President Nixon sent a letter to the Committee urging approval of a plan to set up a Consumer Safety Administration within HEW. However, Arnold B. Elkind, Chairman of the National Commission on Product Safety, came before our Commerce Committee and warned that, if the Administration bill were enacted:

> It would be as though the government were to fashion, like Dr. Frankenstein, a man with beautiful sinews, long arms and piercing eyes, with just one weakness: an inability to hear from the consumer and to respond to his needs.

The Senate Commerce Committee approved the Product Safety Bill on March 24, 1972. It carried the provisions of establishing an independent Consumer Safety Agency with authority over virtually all consumer goods, including food, drugs, and cosmetics. Since the bill would alter the government regulatory process and would affect the life of virtually every American, the Commerce Committee sent the bill to the Senate Government Operations Committee and to the Senate Labor and Public Welfare Committee for their consideration.

These Committees recommended certain changes, such as moving authority for meat, poultry, eggs, and other agricultural product inspection laws over to the Product Safety Agency, and also to transfer to the new agency the authority under the Hazardous Substances Act, the Flammable Fabrics Act, the Radiation Control for Health and

Safety Act, the Poison Prevention Packaging Act, the Refrigerator Safety Act, and the Food, Drug, and Cosmetic Act. These changes should be very helpful to the average consumer, allowing him to come to one independent agency, rather than battle through layer upon layer of bureaucracy.

The Consumer Protection Bill pased the Senate in June 1972, and House action came in September 1972. The vote in the Senate was 69-10. The House was equally strong in its support for the bill with the final roll call vote being 318-50. Since there were differences between the Senate and House, we met several times in late September and early October 1972, and worked out a final measure which was approved by the House on October 13, the Senate on October 14, and signed by the President on October 27, 1972.

The final bill included provisions for transferring to the Commission the functions under the federal Hazardous Substances Act, the Poison Prevention Packaging Act, the Flammable Fabrics Act, and the Refrigerator Safety Act.

A major goal of these transfers were to consolidate all of the consumer-safety regulations within a single agency that would be concerned solely with consumer problems. For example, the Hazardous Substances Act includes toy safety and protection of children. This Act is designed to prevent the use in a toy or household product of any substance that is deemed hazardous because it is toxic, corrosive, an irritant, flammable, or a product that:

> generates pressure through decomposition, heat, or other means, if such substance or mixture of substances may cause personal injury or as a proximate result of any customary or reasonably foreseeable handling or use, including reasonably foreseeable ingestion by children.

This Act allows the new Commission to name any substance as hazardous if it meets this criterion. It requires adequately covering toys that present an electrical, mechanical, or thermal hazard. The Act also indicates that additional labeling may be ordered for a product if the Commission feels that the standard format is not sufficient to inform the public.

When the Commission feels a substance presents an "imminent hazard" to the health and safety of the public, an order may be issued immediately banning the item from sale in interstate commerce.

The Poison Prevention Packing Act sets standards for packaging of household substances that are easily accessible to children and would be harmful to them if handled or ingested. Types of products used around the household that could be subject to special child protection packaging rules include hazardous substances, pesticides, foods, drugs, and cosmetics.

Items covered would be ball point ink cartridges that use toxic ink, cigarette lighters that use butane fuel, charcoal briquets, liquid furniture polish that contains petroleum distillates, liquid preparations that contain wintergreen oil, and household substances that contain such things as sodium hydroxide and turpentine.

The Flammable Fabrics Act reminds me very vividly of the testimony given to us on the Commerce Committee in May 1967 by NBC's nationally known television news correspondent, Peter Hackes. I describe this law and my amendments that were ultimately adopted that year in my book, *The Dark Side of the Marketplace: The Plight of the American Consumer.*

Mr. Hackes' testimony related the story of his daughter, Carol, then 11, who dropped a match onto a cotton blouse which she was wearing.

As Mr. Hackes described it:

It ignited immediately. At first it smoldered, and when she beat at it, it appeared to go out. Momentarily, however, there came a lick of flame which again looked to be out each time she beat it, but within seconds it flared up . . . The events of that day are seared into the minds of my family — and especially into Carol's — like the details of a nightmare.

Carol was burned over 15 percent of her body, from a point

just above the navel to high on the front of her neck, just under her chin. She was hospitalized for nine weeks, and often during that time her parents stood outside her room, listening helplessly to her screams as the doctor administered the painful burn treatments.

The extraordinary part of that story was that the burned blouse was tested and was judged to be perfectly safe under the Flammable Fabrics Act that existed at that time. The legislation to keep hazardous products off the market was spotty, inadequate, and left many products out of safety restrictions. In some cases, even when there were regulations of a product, the standards were so low as to be extremely ineffective.

The new Consumer Product Safety Commission will not be foolproof. No Commission that is created through the tugs and pulls of the legislative process can cover everything. However, this new Commission is clearly a milestone and represents a phenomenal improvement over everything that we have had to date.

Congress usually takes action in response to public demand for protection. The initial Flammable Fabrics Act was passed in 1953, after the country was shocked by deaths and burns from sweaters that went up like torches. In 1956, the pathetic problem of youngsters suffocating inside refrigerators led to the Refrigerator Safety Act. This required that refrigerator doors be made so that they can be opened from the inside. In 1960, we passed the Hazardous Substances Act, which required stringent warnings on all household substances. In 1966, we passed the Child Protection Act, which prohibited the sale of all substances and toys too hazardous for common usage.

But this was only a patchwork quilt that scarcely covered the need for overall safety protection. Americans by and large still remain totally unprotected from vast numbers of potentially injurious and deadly products. This patchwork led us to feel that the only way to approach the problem was to look at the entire range of products in and around the household and establish a comprehensive program. It was through this com-

92

prehensive approach that the initial study commission was established, and their recommendations led to the formation of the Consumer Product Safety Commission.

This Commission is not the final and definitive answer to all the needs of consumers, but is the most extensive protective legislation that has yet been passed by Congress. The potential for such a Commission must now be implemented, and those of us who have worked so long and hard to make sure that this legislation became law will watch the Commission very carefully to ensure that its regulations will do all that we had intended by this legislation. The Consumer Product Safety Commission will be able to develop regulations that require a manufacturer to furnish advance notice and a description of new products, and will have authority to look at product safety rules, ban products that are hazardous, and seek court orders to seize imminently hazardous products.

The greatest attention of this Commission has been given to setting standards, but the broad authority given in the fields of information and research may prove to be just as effective in reducing the incidence of product-caused injuries, deaths, and illnesses.

The Consumer Product Safety Act directs the Commission to maintain an Injury Information Clearinghouse, to conduct continuing investigation of injuries involving consumer products, and to disseminate product safety information to the public. In addition, the Commission is authorized to conduct research and investigations to test products, develop testing methods, and train others in product safety investigation.

Probably the most important function of the Commission in this area will be to collect information on the causes and prevention of product related injuries, and to bring this information to the public. This will form the basis for a consumer education program that could conceivably do more to prevent product related injuries than any of the product safety standards.

There is no easy way to cut down on injuries and accidents around the household. However, Congress has gone a long way toward making a serious impact on these accidents by the creation of this Commission and has thereby taken some long strides in the all-important health area of preventive health. Protecting a child from injury or death caused by an unsafe product is as meaningful as protecting him from disease through immunization.

7.   Research

Scene One: On Saturday, July 31, 1973, Senator Mike Mansfield, the Majority Leader of the United States Senate, and I held a press conference just outside the Senate chambers.

We felt that the situation was so critical as to warrant extraordinary attention. The focus was the serious cutbacks proposed by the Nixon Administration within the health research field. We had just received the results of a massive investigation by the Government Accounting Office (GAO), the investigating arm for Congress, and the Congressional Research Service of the Library of Congress. The results of this investigation convinced Senator Mansfield and me that nothing would suffice short of a major press conference that would alert the rest of Congress and the public at large. The damage from following the administration's proposed course of action would, unless changed, hurt this country for decades. This was brought home to us by the internal documents that GAO uncovered — documents that show that even government scientists did not agree with what the President was trying to do.

Perhaps the most alarming case was made by Dr. Robert Q. Marston, at that time (December 1972) the director of the National Institutes of Health. In a memorandum to the Office of Management and the Budget, Marston implored the President to be aware of what was happening to our health programs. The letter stated in part:

I am sure that you are well aware of the seriousness of the cuts to the NIH program; the impact will be felt for many years to come. While we certainly understand the dimensions of the problem that dictated the fiscal strategy that shaped the HEW budget, the President should be made aware of the long-range impact that this will have to the health of the nation.

A month later, Marston was fired. Apparently the Nixon Administration did not want to hear his opposition to deep budget cuts in the medical research program.

Scene Two: On October 18, 1973, Olympic Hotel, Seattle, Washington, the Albert Lasker Medical Research Awards Dinner took place far from its customary site in New York City. It was also unusual in that it marked one of the few times that the honor was bestowed on a layman rather than a distinguished scientist or physician. It marked the recognition by the research awards jury of the important role that Congress has played in medical research. I was deeply humbled to be chosen as the symbol for Congress in receiving the award.

But the importance of that evening was not in past accomplishments, but in the challenges which lie ahead. A warning for the future was eloquently brought out by Dr. Michael E. DeBakey, world-renowned heart surgeon at Baylor College of Medicine, as he made the results of years of research come alive with the following case study:

When this patient first came to me twenty years ago, he was severely limited in his walking capacity, and the threat of gangrene was imminent because arterial disease was blocking the vessels supplying blood to his feet and legs. Were it not for medical research, we would have had to amputate his legs. Instead, we were able to replace his diseased vessels with artificial arteries, and thus restore normal circulation to his legs. After the operation, he resumed his normal activities in his work as an executive. Since then, I have seen him annually for follow-up examinations, and he has had no more trouble with his legs.

Thirteen years later, the patient returned to the hospital. He was in heart failure from a defective mitral valve. Again, we were able to save his life by applying the fruits of medical research. We replaced his defective valve with an artificial valve, and his heart function returned to normal. Since that time, he has had no evidence of heart failure.

A few years later, the patient returned to see me because of carotid arterial disease. He had had several small strokes as a result of arteriosclerotic occlusion of the carotid arteries supplying blood to the brain. Untreated, his condition would have led to a large stroke that would have caused paralytic disability or possibly death. But again, medical research intervened. We operated on both blocked arteries in his neck, replaced the diseased vessels, and restored normal circulation to his brain. Since then, he has had no further manifestations of stroke.

Three years ago, the patient returned to the hospital because of a massively bleeding ulcer which required partial resection of the stomach. He recovered completely from that operation and resumed his normal activities. This patient is now seventy-four years old, and still leads a useful, happy, productive life as a business executive.

Any one of these serious medical conditions could have led to his permanent disability or even death, and yet each time, we were able to restore his health so that he could lead a normal life, remain economically independent, and continue to be a taxpayer instead of becoming a tax burden. The knowledge used in the effective treatment in each of these conditions came directly from medical research. Without that medical research, this man would not have been able to maintain a responsible position in his community and to make contributions to society throughout the past twenty years.

His case is not, as you might think, unusual or atypical. Because of the new knowledge we have gained from laboratory research, we are able every day to discharge similar patients from the hospital to return to normal living and resume productive, self-sufficient lives. These accomplishments did not, however, occur overnight, notwithstanding press announcements of breakthroughs. Almost every medical advance has come after years of persistent and often tedious efforts of scores of researches. Many frustrations have usually preceded the so-called breakthrough — blind alleys, uncertainties, and disappointments. To be fruitful, research must be pursued with persistence and dedication. We cannot support only the moment of discovery, but must finance all the many months or years of arduous work that precede it.

As much pride as we deserve in our accomplishments, we must not be satisfied to rest on our laurels, for we still have a very long way to go in health. To cite just one statistic, about 23 million Americans still suffer from high blood pressure, some unaware they have the disease. Yet, if untreated, hypertension can result in death from stroke or heart failure. Many other diseases remain inscrutable — not only cancer, but muscular dystrophy, multiple sclerosis, arthritis, cystic fibrosis — the list can be extended considerably. In all of these, we are making progress, but not as rapidly as we could if we were willing to give more financial support to medical research.

This case described by Dr. DeBakey probably sums up as well as anyone could the kind of progress our medical research has made in heart research over the last twenty years. Yet, the Nixon Administration has proposed that we cut back in areas of heart research.

Judith Randal, writing in the *Washington Star-News* on October 18, 1973, looked in depth at documents that were obtained for Senator Mansfield and me through the GAO and

98

Library of Congress investigations that we ordered. The documents were those prepared by the National Heart and Lung Institute (NHLI), a part of the National Institutes of Health. According to these internal reports, projects were in jeopardy which sought to reduce deaths and disability from heart attack by lessening or eliminating the risks posed by the combination of high blood pressure, high blood cholesterol, and cigarette smoking.

A delay in recruitment to enroll patients would lead to an increase in the length of time for this trial, and would result in a greater total cost, said the experts at the Heart and Lung Institute.

"A related project facing a slow-down because of the cut-back of funds," wrote Ms. Randal, "is a cooperative five- to seven-year study among twelve clinics which had planned to find out whether cholystyramine — a cholesterol-lowering drug — would significantly help to reduce heart attacks among men with a common form of blood fat abnormality called hyper-lipidemia type 2 — a subject that is controversial among doctors."

The twelve clinics had already been set up, but the Nixon Administration budget for the fiscal year was not adequate to pay for the drugs, repeated diagnostic tests, and other expenses required for such an effort. The Heart and Lung Institute experts warned that, having funded the clinic, it would be wasteful and inopportune not to start the trial immediately, and pointed out that, in failing to adequately support this and other research efforts, the President faced possible criticism for breaking faith with his own public utterances on the Administration's commitment to the conquest of heart disease.

And that was not all. The litany of program cutbacks in the research area by the Nixon Administration has seemed endless. Another example is in kidney research, where cutbacks threatened to bring about an exorbitant future cost in money and human suffering. Scientists at the National Institutes of Health indicated that the administration had made sharp cutbacks in the agency's request for budget year 1974.

These budget cutbacks came at the very time that the federal government had accepted the obligation to pay the cost of treating Americans of all ages who had kidney disease.

As of July 31, 1973, the Social Security law established that the government would pay most of the cost of artificial kidney treatment or transplantation for patients suffering from incurable kidney disease. The government will be spending over $250 million in 1974 for these programs of kidney treatment. Without any research breakthroughs, this spending will approach $1 billion in the next few years. Dialysis is an artifical kidney treatment that removes wastes from the circulation of the body that a normal kidney would be able to remove without assistance. New technology in this area has led to the development of dialysis machines that will take the place of a normal kidney when something goes wrong. While these artificial kidney machines offer the gift of life to once doomed kidney-disease patients, they are only an interim step to the long-term solution — and they are very costly. Annual cost to a patient may exceed $10,000. It is obvious that new medical breakthroughs are needed to solve the mysteries of kidney disease. Research in this area should be an important auxiliary to the life-saving machines we have developed. As wonderful as they are, no one enjoys the thought of living only through the grace of a machine. There are better answers in the future — if we seek them.

Chronic kidney disease is currently responsible for 55,000 deaths annually in the United States. Approximately 8,000 people are considered suitable for the long-term kidney treatment each year. There is no doubt that basic research must be done in this area, yet the Administration has recommended that kidney research be cut from $17.7 million in budget year 1973 to $15.6 million for budget year 1974.

Most of the kidney research done by the federal government is funded by one of the National Institutes of Health, the National Institute of Arthritis, Metabolism and Digestive Diseases (NIAMDD). This Institute also sponsors a broad range of research in areas such as arthritis, diabetes, and diseases of the digestive tract.

Most of the research that this Institute is doing relates to the problems that we encounter with aging. Yet, the Nixon Administration took the proposed budget of this very important Institute, which was $176.3 million for 1974, and cut it back by $43 million.

Senator Mansfield and I, after the analysis of the General Accounting Office, concluded:

> . . .That this approach is unconscionable, not only from a humanitarian viewpoint of eliminating premature death and disability, but is equally callous from a financial standpoint. Cutting back on kidney research now practically ensures exorbitant future financial outlays and suffering for citizens with end-stage kidney disease.

Scene Three: The United States Senate Subcommittee on Appropriations, on Monday, June 18, 1973, was considering the budget request for Health, Education and Welfare. The topic was the National Institutes of Health. Dr. John F. Sherman was presenting the Administration position, and I was accompanied by two distinguished Republican Senators, Clifford Case of New Jersey and Hiram Fong of Hawaii.

Senator Case used this occasion to obtain the professional judgment of the scientists inside the government on the Nixon Administration proposal to cut out training programs for medical scientists.

Senator Case: I would like to ask you what was your judgment about phasing down training grants and fellowships.

Dr. Sherman: I think it is well known, Senator Case, that over the last three years, NIH has engaged in an effort to review the training grant fellowship programs for the production of bio-medical scientists in an effort to justify their continuation. The position of NIH is

101

	well known; that is, we felt that there could be established a justification for continuation of these programs. There was a decision made at the policy level which went contrary to what NIH had attempted to justify.
Senator Case:	So, in effect, you are phasing out the training grants and fellowship programs.
Dr. Sherman:	Yes, sir.
Senator Case:	And that is because the Administration has decided that there should not be any partiality or special favoritism given to people in the bio-medical field.
Dr. Sherman:	Yes, sir.
Senator Case:	But your experience up to that time has been that, fairness aside, you were producing scientists.
Dr. Sherman:	Yes, sir; the record will show that.

This decision to phase out the training of medical scientists conflicts with the major study done by the National Institutes of Health after a three-year intensive examination of the impact of these training programs.

The major conclusion of the NIH study was that:

Medical research training must be viewed as a subset of the NIH research program. The success, even the viability, of the federal health research effort will depend on the availability of excellent scientists, and a network of institutions of excellence capable of producing superior research manpower.

The chief recommendation of the study was that training biomedical scientists be reinstated as a necessary role for the federal government. Medical research and training programs cannot operate on a haphazard or sporadic basis. Research efforts demand a long lead time in order to be effective.

The problem of cutting back research training grants becomes even more acute when one looks at the results of a questionnaire done by the Association of American Medical Colleges and sent to training fellows at every medical school in the country. Over 4,000 of these fellows were asked: "If no stipend had been available to support your training, but a long-term low interest loan had been available, would you have been able to continue your plans for training?" The answer to this question was "No" from 62 percent of the respondents. It must be remembered that it is this pool of people being trained in research from which future teachers of medicine arrive, both as replacements and for the larger classes of students in the existing schools and in new schools being opened. If we are to train more physicians in this country, it is obvious that we need more teachers than we have. It does not make sense to cut back on the group that will become the teachers of the future.

The primary reason for medical research is to increase the understanding of man and his disorders, and to provide the means for the prevention and treatment of disease.

Dr. DeBakey pointed out some of these breakthroughs in his speech, "Keeping Our World Leadership in Medical Research."

Without exception, the major medical discoveries that have extended the quality and duration of life during the past quarter century can be traced to the research laboratory, whether they be spectacular feats like organ transplantation, or less dramatic discoveries, like drugs to treat epilepsy. The research laboratory gave us vaccines, antibiotics and other miracle drugs that have controlled such previously fatal infections as poliomyelitis, diphtheria, pneumonia, mumps, and measles.

Psychotropic drugs developed in the research laboratory have returned thousands of previously institutionalized patients to a productive place in society. Improved methods of diagnosis and of monitoring the vital signs of patients have greatly aided doctors in ministering to the health of people. Effective medication has reduced the death rate from high blood pressure by 50 percent. Just

103

a decade ago, the incidence of hospital deaths from heart attacks was about 30 percent as compared to a low 6 percent in the best medical centers. Thus, in a short 10 years, we have reduced the death rate by 24 percent, and that reduction is directly attributable to the new knowledge we have gained from medical research.

In my own field of cardio-vascular surgery, the dramatic results of open-heart surgery continue to convert incapacitated patients to happy, useful human beings. Thousands of previously doomed men and women are going about their normal activities today because medical research made possible artifical arteries as a substitute for diseased or worn vessels, and gave us the heart/lung machine to permit surgery directly on the heart to replace malfunctioning valves, to correct congenital anomalies, and more recently, to restore normal coronary arterial circulation. The list of accomplishments of medical research is too long to enumerate, but none of them would have been possible without the support you have given to medical research from your tax dollars.

Dr. DeBakey goes on to point out that these accomplishments did not occur overnight, notwithstanding press announcements of "breakthroughs". Almost every medical advance has come after years of persistent and often tedious effort by scores of researchers. Many frustrations have usually preceded the so-called breakthrough: blind alleys, uncertainties, and disappointments.

To be fruitful, research must be pursued with persistence and dedication. We cannot support only the moment of discovery, but must finance all of the many months or years of arduous work that precede it.

For instance, in the case of infectious or communicable diseases, many common illnesses have either been sharply reduced or eliminated within the last ten or twelve years. Important examples include polio, measles, and rubella. Cures for all of these diseases depended upon discovering the virus, growing it in a tissue culture, and then finding a vaccination that would combat the virus.

Cures for chronic diseases such as cancer are much more complex. Advances in medical research cause us to be both encouraged and excited on one hand, and discouraged and depressed on the other.

For example, we are now told that approximately one-half of all individuals in this country who come down with one form or another of cancer could be treated or the cancer itself could be prevented. The discouraging aspect, however, is that many of the known methods for treatment or prevention are not available to or used by the population. This calls for a much greater effort at public information and at the dissemination of technology to people across our nation.

Better technology and public information will help in the near term future. The long term and more permanent advances will come with laboratory breakthroughs. That is why I question the NIH directors so intensely each year when they appear at our Congressional hearings.

I tried to elicit more information on breakthroughs by having Dr. Rauscher come before our Health Appropriations Subcommittee.

I focused on the viruses causing cancer:

Senator Magnuson: Tell us about the current state of immunization and the traces of viruses found in human cancers.

Dr. Rauscher: Scientists can now identify chemical traces of viruses in human cancers and investigators are learning how to block viral action in the hope that this knowledge can be applied to human cancers. Basic research is being conducted in all the major areas of the biomedical sciences relevant to cancer.

Senator Magnuson: Please go a little further. Tell us about the processes that might work. There are studies going on in immunization, are there not?

Dr. Rauscher: There are studies going on. It is one of the highlights of this year, as a matter of fact. Our major hope is that, when viruses are

105

isolated and proven to cause human cancer, we will be able to make vaccines out of them in the same way that we prevent polio, measles, and so forth. We have an active program in this now.

Senator Magnuson: Does this look promising to you?

Dr. Rauscher: Very promising. It is only one means to prevent cancer. There are problems when one considers vaccines for cancer. Albert Sabin was able to show in only one summer that he had a good vaccine for polio. That is because the disease occurs very shortly after infection. In cancer, it might take as long as seven years to find out whether a vaccine we have today is any good. For example, with acute lymphocytic leukemia in childhood that we hear about, it does not peak until about ages five to seven, so we will probably have to vaccinate during the first year and then wait that long to see how good it is. There might be ways around this. It is all very exciting.

Senator Magnuson: Have any cancer viruses been isolated yet?

Dr. Rauscher: We know of about 120 cancer viruses that cause cancer in animals, including monkeys. We have viruses we call candidates for humans because we have not proved that they cause cancer in humans. They have to do with cancer of the female cervix, the penile region of the male, the postnasal area behind the nose, as well as leukemia and Hodgkin's disease, and possibly bone carcinomas of children.

These are areas where we might have viruses that may be causative. It takes a lot of time and effort to make this proof.

Senator Magnuson: It takes some money too, does it not?

Dr. Rauscher: It takes quite a bit of money.

Senator Magnuson: I think it is important for you to have the wherewithall to move into these important areas of research with vigor. Congress has always been sympathetic to this and I would guess, if you asked the average American what headline he would like to see on any given morning when he wakes up, he would probably suggest in bold type, "Cure for Cancer Found." This is the one I would like to see.

Dr. Rauscher: I agree.

The Senate Health Appropriations Subcommittee has been particularly concerned with health problems of elderly citizens as well as children. In order to learn more about progress in research affecting elderly citizens, we called in Dr. G. Donald Whedon, the Director of the National Institute of Arthritis, Metabolism and Digestive Diseases (NIAMDD), on June 27, 1973. Senator Cotton and I questioned Dr. Whedon about the status of several of the important chronic diseases that his Institute covers.

Dr. Whedon indicated that diabetes has the dubious distinction of being the best known metabolic disease, ranking seventh in the list of diseases causing death in the United States. It affects about 4.5 million Americans, with an additional five million who, by genetic disposition, will develop the disease during their lifetimes.

The goal in diabetes research is understanding the basic impairment of insulin activity. There is equal concern with suppressing the development of the serious vascular and neurological complications of diabetes as well as with better methods of treatment. The Institute will also continue to investigate the wide range of other metabolic diseases, including cystic fibrosis.

There are a number of side effects which may develop for the diabetic patient. These include complications in the kidneys, nervous system, eyes, and the cardio-vascular system.

Modern diabetes research is focused upon finding the cause of the disease by studying insulin, how it is produced and released, and how it does its vital work. Research is also concerned with eliminating the serious blood and nervous system complications that arise.

Although diabetes is probably the most intensively studied of the metabolic diseases, it is hardly the best understood. Advances depend upon further knowledge of the disease and its complications, of genetic factors, and of insulin action.

Senator Cotton: You start off your statement saying that diabetes ranks seventh among killer diseases in the United States, but Chairman Magnuson has noted that you are funding diabetes at $7 million. That is less than the 1972 level. What is the total cost to the economy as a result of this disease? Wouldn't it be money well spent if we increased the research effort instead of lowering it?

Dr. Whedon: Mr. Chairman, the estimated annual cost to the economy of diabetes is $2 billion. This includes $156 million in direct medical costs, and as part of that, there is an estimated $50 million for the oral drugs, and then the remainder of the $156 million is in insulin, syringes, and other equipment. There are 35,000 deaths per year from diabetes, and the incidence is estimated to be about 325,000 new cases per year.

1973 was a very important year for NIAMDD. Dr. Christian B. Anfinsen, an NIH scientist, won a Nobel Prize in chemistry for his pioneering work in enzymes. This work is very important in understanding abnormalities in the makeup of proteins. Also, Dr. Gerald M. Edelman, of Rockefeller University, a grant-supported scientist from NIAMDD, was awarded a Nobel Prize in physiology and medicine for his work on immunology. This work is basic to many diseases, including rheumatoid arthritis.

Dr. Whedon indicated that arthritis and rheumatism head the list of chronic diseases in the United States today in terms of social and economic importance. Research energies here must focus on developing a clear understanding of the underlying mechanism of the diseases. NIAMDD will attempt to identify a virus and determine the immune system malfunction which seems to lead to rheumatoid arthritis.

Arthritis and rheumatism refer to the swelling and the breakdown of joints and to diseases affecting the tissues around the joints. These chronic diseases lead the country in terms of social and economic importance. They inflict much suffering and disability on over 17 million Americans and cost the economy about $4 billion a year.

One scientist has reported preliminary success in some rheumatoid patients with severely inflamed joints by injecting a drug into the affected joints. These drug dosages were experimental, but this is promising work and should be studied closely.

Another promising area is in total knee-joint replacement. To date more than 300 knee-joints damaged by arthritis have been replaced. NIH reports that the relief of pain and resumption of basic daily activities previously denied by this disability are sufficiently encouraging that this development in orthopedic surgery merits consistent support.

As in kidney disease, mechanical devices are only an interim answer. The Institute feels that its research energies must be focused on developing a clear understanding of the underlying causes of rheumatism. Until that goal is achieved, it is unlikely that there will be effective methods of prevention, control, or cure of arthritis. To meet that end, the Institute has directed research toward identifying a possible virus and toward discovering the specific malfunctions of the immune system of the body.

The state of research here seems to fit Dr. DeBakey's description that before there are breakthroughs there must be years of persistent, often tedious efforts by scores of researchers.

In examining these important chronic diseases, two major points can be made. The annual cost to the nation of arthritis is close to $9 billion. Over $700 million is lost each year in taxes that would have been paid to federal, state, and local governments. In terms of priorities, $14 million was proposed for research in the arthritis area. It is not enough. It amounts to only seven cents a year for every American citizen, yet, the per capita cost of arthritis each year is $43.70. I do not like to bandy about statistics and numbers, but seven cents for pervention, compared to $43.70 in losses, is outrageous. And these figures do not even reflect the pain and grief. The old adage of an ounce of prevention saves a pound of cure seems to be most appropriate in this regard.

Many scientists and experts have warned that we should only discuss the "success" stories of research, for fear of alarming or disappointing the public. Arthritis is certainly not a success story, in spite of the progress described above. For too many of the poor victims of arthritis, in spite of all the research, the best treatment is still only aspirin to alleviate some of the pain.

The public understands the difficulties of coming up with easy solutions. Furthermore, it recognizes that disappointing results in new treatments for arthritis have to be balanced by exciting new treatments for such diseases as childhood leukemia.

There has been remarkable progress in just the last few years in dealing with childhood leukemia. Once absolutely and universally fatal, it can now in many instances be controlled. Research in this area has enabled scientists to better design drug doses and schedules to help control the growth of leukemia cells. Although science does not yet understand how these cancer cells grow, the development of these anti-leukemic drugs has helped in dealing with patients. This kind of clinical research, combined with drug study research, has formed the basis of the substantial advances that have been made in the past decade.

Progress in this area has not been easy. Research first found that several drugs were able to cause a remission (a temporary stopping of the cancer growth). But these remissions were invariably followed by a relapse, and would often lead to problems with the nervous system. Scientists, through long, tedious and methodical research, have now found a combination of drugs that can overcome most of these problems. As a result, the incidence of remission in childhood leukemia is more than 90 percent and the remissions that have been obtained are greatly prolonged. Only ten years ago, it was a rare child with leukemia who lived as long as five years. Today, more than 50 percent of these youngsters live at least five years.

While this is not the ultimate solution, it is certainly a tribute to the scientists in this country to have brought about this kind of progress. It is my opinion that such results make all the money which we have invested in medical research worth the effort.

As successful as scientists have been with childhood leukemia, there are other children's diseases that will require extensive research before cures are even on the horizon.

Early in 1973, in a small California town, John and Patricia Smiley went into the bedroom of their four year old infant. The child, healthy the day before, lay dead. The couple, frantic with sudden shock, immediately called the local Sheriff's office to ask for an ambulance. As Smiley remembers it, the voice at the other end replied that, if the child was dead, why was an ambulance needed?

So began the post-dealth ordeal of the Smileys. This couple, both young and poor, were charged on suspicion of involuntary manslaughter. They were jailed for three days! The charges were eventually dropped, but not before the couple had been harrassed to the point that they left town.

John Smiley told his story to the Senate Committee on Labor and Public Welfare in September 1973:

There are just so many bad memories to the whole situation, and I would like to forget. But I know that I

111

will never be able to. I hope that it never happens to anyone else like it happened to us. The death of a child is bad enough. It's the harrassment and lack of knowledge, lack of understanding, the lack of compassion that hurts more than anything else.

Between 10,000 and 15,000 children die each year in the United States, victims of the sudden infant death syndrome (SIDS), or "crib death." This disease is now one of medicine's most serious, unsolved mysteries.

It is a disease that kills more infants between the ages of one month and one year than any other disease. It is second only to accidents as the most frequent cause of death for children under 15. Twice as many children die each year of crib death as die of cancer.

Crib death always occurs during sleep, but is apparently not predictable nor preventable, nor is it new. Authorities on crib death find references to the tragedy in the Bible, "overlaying" is described, the theory at that time being that mothers who slept with their infants rolled over and suffocated or crushed them.

In 1892, an Edinburg medical journal carried an article by a Scottish physician in which the disease was erroneously attributed to suffocation.

The typical case is a mother who puts her baby to bed with no suspicion that anything is wrong. The infant dies during the night. An autopsy may reveal minor inflammation of the respiratory tract, and some congestion of the lungs, but these conditions are not found to be severe enough to cause death.

A major difficulty with this disease is the mystery of the unexpected, seemingly unexplainable death of an unattended child. The public is uninformed about this strange ailment. Law enforcement officials, the community at large, and even health professionals suspect criminal neglect, and do not treat the parents as individuals who are grieving over the death of a loved infant. On the contrary, they often heap more guilt on top of the unjustified guilt felt by the parents.

Dr. Abraham Bergman of Children's Orthopedic

112

Hospital and Medical Center in Seattle is President of the National Foundation for Sudden Infant Deaths, Inc., and is also a good personal friend. He indicates that six cases were brought to his attention in 1973 alone where parents were thrown in jail. Even when such severe action is not taken, the investigators often end up asking such questions as, "How many times did you hit the baby?", "Did your other child choke or in any way abuse the baby?", or "Did you let your dog bite the baby?" Is it any wonder that families that suffer this tragedy live for months and sometimes years with torment over the death of their baby and often become candidates themselves for psychotherapeutic help?

Even when the investigating officials seem compassionate, the mental torment and anguish is still there, often caused by ignorance and unsympathetic health officials.

The following letter sent by a New York State resident to the National SIDS Group describes the problem most vividly:

Dear Sirs:

I am very interested in helping your organization with public awareness of the different aspects of sudden infant death.

I have followed the Senate investigation through the news media, but I want to do something about it. My first son (my only son) was born on August 26, 1966. He weighed seven pounds, eight ounces, was 21 inches long, and was just fine. A week later, my neighbor gave birth to a girl. It was a joke of how they would probably be sweethearts. Both babies prospered. In November 1966, my girl friend's baby was found dead in her crib, a victim of crib death. I was so stunned I couldn't think of words to comfort the parents, who were my friends. The next Thursday was Thanksgiving.

At home, no one talked much about the "lost baby", but rather of the parents.

Sunday, November 27, 1966, we all slept late. I got breakfast ready and went upstairs to get the children. Tracy, age 15 months, was wide awake in her crib; I glanced over at my son's crib, and he was still sleeping. I brought Tracy downstairs and put her in her high chair, set her breakfast in front of her, and went to get my husband up. He sat down at the kitchen table, I poured him coffee and went upstairs to bring my son down. I looked at him and he seemed so peaceful. I began to pick him up and his hand was limp. I looked at his face — one side was white, the other was blue. I screamed for my husband, and we shook him and nothing! I ran downstairs and called the police (we lived in a small town of 1,500 people). The policeman didn't ask any questions, he picked up my son and began to give him mouth-to-mouth resuscitation. The police chief came in and asked us for our pediatrician's name and phone number. The doctor was in a town some fifteen miles away, and of course, no one could reach him. There were three doctors in our town, but none of them would come to our house. The chief called for an ambulance with first aid team. It took a half an hour. As they pulled in with their oxygen, I had hope. The police chief asked us a few questions regarding the health of the baby and the circumstances regarding him and how I found him. I was terrified. I answered the questions, but I knew they would think I did something to him.

The oxygen brought color into his face, and I felt sure that he would live. The ambulance men were going to take him to the nearest hospital, which is eighteen miles away. Just as they carried him out to the ambulance, our family dentist came over with a bag to see if he could help. He was the only doctor willing to help, and he advised us to go to the hospital.

As we got to the emergency room door of the hospital, we could see the ambulance backing in.

Two weeks later, a baby at the other end of town died the same way, and all three babies are all buried together.

I couldn't really thank the police for their help. They were wonderful, but the doctors involved, as well as the pathologist and the medical examiner, should have been brought before some board of inquiry, as to why they wouldn't come to our house, and why they kept questioning over and over again.

It took me five years to decide to have another baby; plus, I left my husband and remarried. We kept blaming each other, and it got worse. In September 1971 I had another baby girl. The first three or four months were hard; I couldn't bear to go into her room to check on her.

Even though I have changed my entire lifestyle, I still have the nightmares and the eerie feeling in my heart. If I only knew why? How could this happen? What causes this?

Please help me to get involved in this.

(Signed) Buffalo, New York

There has been little research into crib death. This has been because there have been too few scientists studying the disease, and only a very small amount of money has been allocated for its research. The causes of crib death are still totally unknown. The only thing that we know for sure is that is a disease and not a crime, and should be treated that way. Medical research seems to be divided over the causes at this point. Dr. Bergman theorizes that crib death occurs because of a sudden closure of the vocal cords during sleep which shuts off the infant's airway. He thinks that the presence of viral infection may make the child vulnerable to the spasm. Other researchers agree that a virus infection may lead to crib death, but think that the heart may also be involved.

Senators Edward Kennedy of Massachusetts and Walter Mondale of Minnesota have been leading the struggle to convince the Nixon Administration that important areas such as this deserve research priority. Dr. Bergmann summed up many of the social factors which his statement to the Senate Subcommittee:

The fact that survivors of crib death victims in the United States are treated like criminals is a national disgrace. With our present state of knowledge, crib death itself is neither predictable nor preventable. The divorces, the mental illnesses, the torment of unrelieved guilt are completely preventable . . . by the humane handling of infant death cases.

Senate bill S. 1745 reached the Senate floor on December 11, 1973. At that time, under the leadership of Senators Kennedy and Mondale, the bill passed the Senate calling for the authorization of $7 million in 1974, $8 million in 1975, and $9 million in 1976 for medical research into the sudden infant death syndrome. There is no doubt that we are a long way from answers about the causes, let alone the cures, of diseases such as arthritis, SIDS, cancer, kidney malfunctioning and others. But with an annual government budget of $304 billion, is it not reasonable to invest at least $7 million in SIDS or more than $14 million into arthritis in order to begin to get some answers? How can reasonable men think otherwise?

8.   Standards and Quality

The *New York Times,* November 27, 1973, carried a United Press International story describing a surgeon in a Sacramento, California hospital who admitted performing at least 37 unnecessary back operations. In ruling that a former patient now dying of cancer be paid $3.7 million in damages, the Superior Court judge said that Dr. N. had performed the operations "with evil purpose . . . simple to line his pockets." Dr. N., who had 25 additional malpractice cases pending against him, and had lost $500,000 judgments in two previous suits, testified that, from 1963 to 1970, he was addicted to "uppers and downers", and admitted performing unnecessary and negligent surgery.

Superior Court Judge Goldberg, in issuing his 196-page decision, termed the case "a five-month horror. The drama played out here was not a fantasy contrived to satisfy a casual fancy for morbid amusement; it was real, permanent, and tragic."

"Here have come the poor, the maimed, and the halt to testify against their once-beloved physician for the wrongs that he committed against them with evil purpose." said Judge Goldberg. "The defendant for nine years made a practice of performing unnecessary surgery and performing it badly, simply to line his pockets."

This story should clearly be viewed as an aberrant horror and far from the mainstream of good American medicine. However, it is quite disturbing that a situation like this could

117

occur at all, not in a private office or in some remote hinterland, but in a hospital in the capital city of one of our largest states.

Dr. Gerber, a Board-certified surgeon, tells a much more sophisticated version of the same tale in his well-known book, *The Gerber Report*.

In a comfortable bed in a modern, sunny room, in a fully accredited hospital, lies Mrs. Molly Jones, who has just had her uterus removed. The service is good, the nurses are cheerful and helpful, and her doctor is the most solicitous of her feelings and welfare. The Jones family has no money, so Mrs. Jones' care will be paid for by Medicaid. Only a few years ago, she would have had to go to the despised county hospital. Now she is getting 'mainstream' medical care, the same that would be rendered to anyone who could pay.

On the floor below Mrs. Jones, in the immaculate, bustling Pediatrics Section of the hospital is little Tommy Brown, who has just surrendered his tonsils. Tommy's family has no money either, yet he too is receiving mainstream care. The stigma of charity medicine is gone; it is indeed a happy picture.

Or is it? It might be, except for one disturbing fact; neither Mrs. Jones nor little Tommy needed the operation. Mrs. Jones' uterus and Tommy's tonsils were perfectly healthy, Both patients have undergone unnecessary pain and suffering in each case at some risk of life. Each is worse off than he was before, at least to that extent. Both occupy beds that are needed by seriously ill patients. The taxpayer will have paid out sizable sums that were totally wasted. The only persons who benefit are the doctors who collect fees for having performed the operation.

You may think that this is an exceptional incident. It is not. It occurs hundreds of times in this country every day.

The examples above raise serious questions about health care, with respect to both quality and accessibility. We are now at the early stage of a broad movement to develop government standards to help protect the consumer. Initial efforts were directed toward rapidly rising costs, but now the questions of delivery of care, the quality of services provided, and the manpower and facilities necessary to provide good care are all being examined.

Health service is in some ways following in the footsteps of air and water pollution control programs which have been recently enacted. The Consumer Product Safety Commission is another result of Congressional feeling that standards must be established in order to protect the average product-buying American.

Most people would argue that it is reasonable, and many that it is overdue, for the government to take a good hard look at making sure that the large amount of money that is being dispersed for medical services is being spent well. As was pointed out in Chater two, the federal health dollar expenditure in direct care services has increased to approximately $25 billion in budget year 1974.

In the past three years, the federal government has become involved in setting health standards in two ways. First, through the Economic Stabilization Program, there has been a period of mandatory cost controls. During Phase IV of this program, health regulations broadened control of costs even in the quantity of medical services provided in a given health-care institution.

Second, a national system of Professional Standards Review Organizations (PSRO) was established to regulate the quality of federally-financed health care. Basically, this program allows organized medicine the opportunity to police the quality and cost of medical care delivered by their fellow physicians.

The consumer should be well aware that establishing standards or regulations alone does not guarantee much improvement. In fact, I have been extremely disturbed by the bureaucratic "red tape" that the Nixon Administration has chosen to impose upon doctors, hospitals, and insurance payers. I have become worried that the people in HEW have been ordered to spend so much time creating new forms that they have not paid enough attention to medical research, training programs, etc.

There is probably nothing as frustrating to a hard-working doctor than to have to spend hours filling out forms and consuming time that could be used caring for patients. This over-obsession with red tape hurts the patients as well. I believe this time could be much better used to emphasize preventive health care and consumer health education.

Congress has gotten more involved in regulating health care through the establishment of regional authorities now being proposed for extensions and replacements of the Hill-Burton hospital construction program, regional medical programs, health maintenance organizations, and comprehensive health planning organizations.

John K. Iglehart, writing for the *National Journal* in November 1973, examined the situation and concluded that government regulation in the health field was not a new phenomenon and was clearly growing.

States have traditionally played the largest role in regulating health care institutions and providers, and this is as it should be. But just as in the areas of air and water pollution and consumer product safety, when it is apparent that national needs and interstate concerns must be protected, then it is appropriate for the federal government to establish certain types of standards. This era of growing consumerism and the need for greater consumer protection, has brought greater awareness of problems such as public health. One concern, of course, is the rapidly growing percentage of income and federal dollars being devoted to medical care. There are other concerns, such as providing the consumer with more information about where care can be had, how to measure its quality, and how to gauge its appropriateness. This is especially true because a number of problems these days are not purely medical, but ethical, legal and social as well. For example, the prior chapter on research points out how unevenly the fruits and accomplishments of medical

120

research get passed on to the general public. It is of equal importance that many advances in technology do not reach practicing physicians rapidly enough either. Many medical experts have told us in Congress that medical knowledge is advancing at the rate of five to eight percent each year. That could mean that a practicing physician who did not keep up with these advances for seven or eight years might be providing care that was 50 percent obsolete in terms of new methods. This has led many experts to advocate that we should be interested in requiring relicensing and proficiency testing of physicians and other health practitioners every so often. I would have to study this much further, but Dr. Claude E. Welch, a Boston surgeon and President of the American College of Surgeons, has predicted that relicensing and recertification of physicians will be required within the decade. He stated that:

Medical knowledge doubles within a decade and . . . senescence occurs more quickly in medical practice than in any other profession.

Recertification or relicensing of health practitioners is only one proposal that is currently being discussed for meeting our health manpower needs. The key question seems to be whether voluntary incentives programs will be sufficient to get adequate manpower distribution. This distribution must not only be in terms of numbers of physicians and other practitioners, but also in terms of the right kinds of specialties. For example, even those individuals who mistakenly argue that we already have enough physicians in this country will concede that their distribution by geography and by specialty is not adequate to serve large portions of our population. If organized medicine, probably through the American Medical Association or the medical schools, does not take steps to alleviate this maldistribution through some voluntary mechanism, then the federal government has no alternative but to establish sanctions to rectify the situation. The medical schools, which have been receiving a large amount of federal aid, are particularly vulnerable to these sanctions.

State governments have moved most rapidly in the last

five or so years to establish programs of cost regulation, particularly aimed at curbing inflation in hospitals. One of the main causes for this activity has been the frequency with which Blue Cross has had to seek rate increases. The second important reason has been the frequency with which state budgets ran into the red because of the Medicaid program.

Generally, state laws have included a "certificate of need" clause, which allows them to approve plans for new medical construction. Other state laws have gone to the extent of empowering an agency to set rates that would be paid to health facilities by the state agencies and by Blue Cross. Other states, such as Connecticut, have in effect created a social or public utility for health care by requiring all health-care institutions to submit a proposed operating budget to the state regulatory commission for approval.

If one looks at developments both at the state and federal levels, one major force seems to be left out, namely, a role for the consumers. This is particularly true in the Professional Standards Review Organizations (PSRO), where physicians have the opportunity to review payment requests of their follow practitioners but consumers lack similar privileges. This omission is particularly important in viewing the future of PSROs, since many assume that they will go beyond monitoring the cost of care now rendered in Medicare and Medicaid to become the mechanism for reviewing the quality of care under a new national health insurance program.

One important question is whether the government will have to attach some minimum standards of care to the reimbursement programs. Many feel that the establishment of PSROs now gives organized medicine the opportunity to provide quality, accessible care. If they are not up to the task, then it is likely that Congress would have to establish the standards necessary to protect the health care consumer.

Health is one of the most difficult areas for the consumer to judge if he is getting his money's worth, because the decision to purchase various kinds of care is often not made by the consumer himself, but by some outside party, usually his physician.

Herbert F. Denenberg, while Insurance Commissioner for the State of Pennsylvania, published a *Shopper's Guide to Hospitals,* intended as a first step in giving the public information it is entitled to have about hospitals. Commissioner Denenberg indicated that:

Much of this information is supposed to be public information, but nonetheless, it has often not been available or has not been publicized, despite its usefulness. For example, many of our hospitals have non-conforming beds that do not meet safety standards.

This information is included in the guide. Such a shopper's guide could reveal the cost of running a hospital and how well that hospital keeps its beds filled. This lets a patient know that he shouldn't have to wait for a bed in a hospital if there are many empty beds, and if there are, that in one way or another, the patients using that institution will have to bear the cost of those beds. There is also the tendency of some hospitals to keep patients longer in order to keep beds filled.

Commissioner Denenberg points out another value of this type of a guide:

Although shopping for a hospital may not be in vogue, greater dissemination of information and wide public awareness might contribute to more hospital economy, especially if the public begins to question costs that appear to be out of line with what others are charging. The public may not be in a position to shop for a hospital, especially in view of a doctor's requirement and his hospital connection. But a consumer is entitled to information that will permit comparisons.

There is other information that could be made available to the public. For example, hospitals are currently rated and approved by the Joint Commission on Accreditation of Hospitals (J.C.A.H.). This rating by the Commission is generally accompanied by a series of comments, including an evaluation of deficiencies and other suggestions to the hospital for improvement. Making this information generally

123

available would allow those interested in improving their local facility to know what the experts feel should be done.

It should be reasonable to expect that a hospital through its Board of Directors will have an established policy on human experimentation and that this policy be made public. It would also seem reasonable that the institution include in its policy statement the right of patients to receive counseling if they are to be involved in human experimentation.

On February 6, 1973, the House of Delegates of the American Hospital Association approved "A Patient's Bill of Rights." The American Hospital Association felt that such a statement would contribute to more effective patient care and greater satisfaction for the patient, his physician, and the hospital organization. One of the statement's twelve provisions is:

> The patient has the right to obtain from his physician complete current information concerning his diagnosis, treatment, and prognosis in terms the patient can be reasonably expected to understand.

Another of the items is:

> The patient has the right to refuse treatment to the extent permitted by law, and to be informed of the medical consequences of his action.

Furthermore:

> The patient has the right to expect that all communications and records pertaining to his care should be treated as confidential.

That the patient's records remain confidential is extremely important, especially since a Medical Information Bureau has been set up by certain private insurance companies, where dossiers are kept on patients without their knowledge.

The American Hospital Association statement indicates that the patient has a right to obtain information as to the professional relationships among individuals, by name, who are treating him.

In April 1973, the Pennsylvania Insurance Department issued its own citizen's bill of hospital rights, because the department felt that the American Hospital Association program, although well intentioned, did not go far enough. The Pennsylvania statement indicated:

> What patients need and must have a right to is quality care at prices they can afford.

This statement recognizes the rights of a citizen regarding hospitals, whether or not he is a patient. Every member of the public pays for hospitals through his health insurance, his Blue Cross and Blue Shield premiums, and his tax dollars, so the bill of rights should apply to all citizens, and not just to patients.

We often hear statements that the hospital directors run the hospitals, or the doctors run the hospitals, or the administrators run the hospitals. Indeed, if hospitals are community hospitals and are non-profit institutions licensed by the states, then the public ought to have more say in what happens, and ought to begin asserting the citizen's existing rights and developing new ones.

To this extent, there should be disclosure by these institutions that allows for public interest and public accountability.

For example, a patient should have the right to file a complaint against the institution, and to have that grievance considered and redressed, if necessary, in a satisfactory and reasonable fashion. This may require that there be a patient advocate to represent the interests of the patient. It is also reasonable to expect that a hospital should agree to go to arbitration for certain types of disputes that are not easily reconciled.

The consumer has a right to know the membership of the Board of Directors, including occupations and major interests of the members of the Board. A community hospital should be run so that the consumer has a voice in the management and planning of the hospital.

The consumer has a right to information about the finances and activities of the hospital, which should include general information about assets, expenses, costs, profit, charges and occupancy. Information should also include the physicians who are on the hospital staff, and the rules and regulations which physicians must apply in their conduct with a patient.

The citizen's bill of hospital rights prepared by the Pennsylvania Insurance Department also includes two very important sections, one concerning access to information concerning records, and a second on consumer advocacy. These declare that:

> The patient has a right to full information about his stay, including information about his bill and access to his hospital records. This includes detailed information about his bill, including itemized charges. This information should be readily available, regardless of the patient's source of payment.
>
> The public has a right to expect a hospital to behave as a consumer advocate, rather than as a business headquarters for doctors and hospital officials. The hospital should affirmatively and aggressively move to protect the patient and his interests rather than rubber-stamp the demands of doctors. The hospital should provide leadership in improving health care for the community.
>
> Hospitals have often had only one idea for changing the health delivery system: getting more money for the hospitals. The hospital is a repository of great know-how and expertise, and should use that know-how responsibly. It should come up with sound proposals for reform, and aggressively advocate the consumer's interests.

The public's very recent feeling that they should be more concerned about the health insurance industry has been partly due to the rapidly growing cost of health insurance, including Blue Cross, in the last few years. In the past, the attitude of the public seemed to be that, if the insurance company was paying for it, the cost didn't really make much difference. However, with costs of care going up so fast, and the insurance companies building in more and more deductibles and co-insurance, and finding other ways for the consumer to share the risk with the insurance company, the public has become more enlightened and more concerned about what is going on.

It has not been easy, however, for individuals to get useful information about their insurance and what they are covered for and what they are not.

Commissioner Denenberg feels:

> The commercial health insurance companies not only do little to improve the health delivery system, but often aggravate existing problems.
>
> This fact is demonstrated by the "junk" insurance, the "gimmick" insurance, and the "Mickey Mouse" insurance which has recently flooded the market as a result of activities of mail-order husksters.

It seems that the attitude of the mail-order insurance industry toward the consumer is to tell as little as necessary and hope that he never finds out the truth.

> Essentially, these firms mask or misrepresent their coverage. In bold headlines, they guarantee a large amount, such as $50,000 in medical expenses, but the fine print negates almost any possibility of claimants receiving more than a fraction of what is being dangled before them.
>
> Insurance is confusing enough for a well-informed person, and even the most sophisticated and educated person is often confused and baffled by all the possibilities. Those in our society who are most vulnerable, such as elderly and low-income individuals, are often led to believe by this advertising that they cannot afford to be without health insurance, and since they are not likely to be eligible for a group insurance contract, such as through an employer, they find that mail-order insurance is about the only type available to them.

Company X has mastered the "bonanza" technique. Headlines scream that the company offers $50,000 in benefits, but what it really offers is about $20 a day if you are in a hospital. Stay sick long enough, and in a hospital, not at home and not at a nursing home, and you will undoubtedly collect your $50,000. Long enough in this case is about five years of continuous hospitalization, a virtual impossibility — and one, needless to add, that would cost far more than the $50,000 promised.

Company X doesn't worry much about a person who might require a long hospital stay, since only 2 percent of all hospitalized people stay longer than 30 days.

What is the average claim paid by this company? $175! What was the largest pay-out? $10,000! This is all a far cry from the advertising which states in bold headlines, "Coverage for $50,000."

There are generally, other restrictions and limitations that such mail-order companies place on their coverage in order not to pay out benefits. For example, there is usually a provision barring payment of benefits until the claimant has been hospitalized for more than seven days. Since the average stay in a hospital is about eight days, then about half the people who enter the hospital and hold one of these policies would never be reimbursed at all. The other major clause that allows the insurance company to get out of paying is the so-called "pre-existing condition" exclusion. In Chapter One, the 50-year-old female whose claim for congestive heart failure was rejected because of "pre-existing" obesity is an example of this gimmick. Some companies even go so far as to build in restrictions on specific diseases, barring coverage if they are discovered during the first six months of coverage. The list is often so inclusive that there is scarcely a disease left out.

Another major problem with mail-order insurance companies is that they generally pay only for hospitalization. This continues to perpetuate a care system that often forces people into the hospital when they need not receive such expensive care.

The Senate Antitrust and Monopoly Subcommittee indicated that one company, National Liberty Corporation, turned an after-tax profit of 27 percent on shareholder equity in 1970, three times that of American Telephone and Telegraph and the Chase Manhattan Bank. In general, these insurance companies do not pay back in benefits more than 50 percent of every dollar that a person pays in insurance premiums. The ultimate for these companies is to sell "dread disease" policies where it has been documented that an insurance company can return to the public as little as seven cents on the dollar.

No one in our population today is more terrified of the prospect of a major illness than the elderly. They must depend upon pensions and Social Security — and a sudden sickness calling for a long hospital stay may eradicate any budgets and savings built up over the years.

Mail-order insurance promoters emphasize that a person needs to supplement his Medicare coverage. What is in small print and not in the advertisement is that these companies pay only a small amount on a daily basis, and then they only begin to pay after the insured person puts out some money himself as a deductible and is in the hospital sixty days under Medicare.

The consumer has the right to know much more about these mail-order insurance firms. The public has to be made aware that some policies that have a premium of one dollar jump substantially after the first month. Also, claims about very high benefits such as $50,000 should be accompanied by a statement that the consumer would have to be in a hospital bed for five years to get this amount of return. The public should also be guaranteed that if an advertisement is endorsed by a famous person, payments for the testimonial or financial interest in the company by that famous person would be acknowledged prominently in the advertisement.

The policies should be made plain enough to be understood and should explain fully the exemptions, limitations, and exclusions that are in the policy. The consumer has the right to be given an honest picture of the kind of insurance that is being sold to him. Such rights have been outlined and guaranteed in a string of consumer-protection bills passed by my Commerce Committee.

The public has a right to be protected and served well and fairly by the health insurance industries. These companies communicate by mail and telephone with millions of Americans, and should be sensitive to the wants and needs of these consumers. The mail-order insurance industry offers accident and health insurance geared largely to supplement a regular basic health insurance program. This fact should be made clear to the public. In addition, such policies limit benefits to their holders. The pre-existing condition provision, for example, should be carefully explained to the public. Consumers have a right to know that most policies include diseases that are not covered for at least the first two years that one makes premium payments. The fact that outside hospital care (outpatient care) is not covered by most of these policies should also be made clear.

The conclusion here becomes inescapable: there has to be some kind of standard form that protects the consumer and allows him to know what he is getting. This does not necessarily mean that mail-order health insurance is all bad or must be eliminated; it merely means that the consumer has a right to know about gaps and deficiencies before he gets sick and not after the bill is rejected by the insurance company. For example, National Liberty Corporation received 78,500 claims during 1970, 1971, and a portion of 1972. Of these claims, 30,000 or nearly 40 percent were rejected and nothing paid. Nearly one-half of the 30,000 rejected claims were due to pre-existing health conditions. When such an extraordinarily high number of claims is rejected, one is hard pressed to come to any conclusion other than that consumers do not really know what is in their insurance policies.

The following was taken from testimony before the Subcommittee on Antitrust and Monopoly of the Senate Judiciary Committee on June 6, 1972. The exchange is between a Senate counsel and the insurance president.

Senate Counsel. This is your file no. 5523546. Now, this person is a 72-year old male who was interred in the hospital from January 12, to January 20, 1972 for replacement of a pacemaker due to failure of the old pacemaker, accompaning an increasing pulse rate. The claim was rejected on the basis of pre-existing condition, as the physician claims it was a condition that existed since 1968.

Here is a man who is functioning normally and will need a new pacemaker like you would need a new dental bridge if your bridgework were out. Yet you denied this claim on the grounds that the condition had existed since 1968.

This man was paying premiums for 15 months. What is your reaction to this kind of insurance?

Insurance Company President. Here is a man who had a condition existing at least four years prior to the time of the claim.

Senate Counsel. Coronary condition, but not a pacemaker condition.

Insurance Company President. Well, I think we are being technical. He would not have the pacemaker if he did not have the coronary problem.

Senate Counsel. On what basis was it denied, denied because of a coronary or on the basis of the facts that the pacemaker wore out and he needed a new pacemaker?

Insurance Company President. Well, if the claim was made because he was in the hospital, it was denied because the condition that

131

existed and the reason he was
in the hospital were pre-
existing at the time that the
policy was taken out.

It might be appropriate to conclude this discussion with
an interchange between Senator Philip Hart of Michigan and
Mr. Leslie T. Hemry, President of the Health Insurance
Association of America, at a Senate hearing in June 1972.
Senator Hart is one of the leading advocates of consumer
protection in the United States Senate and had just completed
an extensive investigation into the commercial health and
accident insurance industry. It should be noted that the
Health Insurance Association of America (HIAA) is an
organization that consists of 326 insurance companies and is
responsible for over 80 percent of the health insurance written
by insurance companies in the United States today.

Senator Hart.   What is your opinion as to the role the mail-
                  order business should play?
Mr. Hemry.   Well, as has been covered many times in the
                  hearings, these plans in general provide
                  supplementary benefits. So long as the public
                  understands that these are not substitutes for
                  basic coverage or comprehensive coverage and
                  all the advertisements and all the sales pitches
                  are honored and the people can understand
                  them, then we see no reason why they should
                  not be permitted to continue.
Senator Hart: I won't be unkind by asking you the name of
                  the company that meets the test you just
                  described, unless you want to volunteer one.
Mr. Hemry.   I think as a trade association person that I
                  appreciate your understanding.

9.　　　　　　　　　　　Manpower and Facilities

Sufficient manpower and adequate facilities are essential to meet the nation's health needs. These resources are necessary in order to get medical care to citizens.

The current health manpower policies provide no meaningful way to supply underserved areas. In fact, the Nixon Administration proposed as recently as May 1974 that financial support for increasing the numbers of doctors be phased out.

The Administration has also proposed that some existing facilities be shut down. The abortive attempt to close the Public Health Service hospitals is an example of that policy.

The Nation's Health, the official newspaper of the American Public Health Association, has a monthly column, "Commentary." The October 1973, column was written by Vernon E. Wilson, M.D., Professor of Community Health and Medical Practice at the University of Missouri at Columbia. Its headline read: "Closing of PHS Hospitals to Prove More Costly In End."

The article was particularly significant because Dr. Wilson had only a short time before served as the Administrator of the Health Services and Mental Health Administration (HSMHA) of HEW. In that capacity he had been involved in the Nixon Administration's call for the closing of the PHS hospitals. Some of us in Congress have been fighting this ill-conceived plan since December 1970.

Dr. Wilson's article had the following to say on this issue:

Among the recent actions taken by the Executive Branch

133

of the federal government, none more clearly portrays the current poverty of concern and understanding for health issues than the proposal to close the Public Health Service hospitals.

Although submitted to Congress as a plan, the proposal vividly represents a political decision, deliberately misrepresented as a plan. The long-standing desire of the Office of Management and Budget (OMB) to destroy these institutions is now being relentlessly pursued without regard for cost to the beneficiaries or the trainees, or the effect upon some important research activities. The lack of either willingness or perhaps capacity on the part of the Executive Branch to understand the implications of this action is more disturbing than the proposal itself.

At the base of the difficulty lies the fact that never before have decisions in PHS had so little health professional input. Admittedly, the executive branch must be politically responsive to the demand for reduced expenditures, but that constitutes an inadequate reason for professional vagrancy.

This venomous attack upon the Administration is not at all unique. Several health experts have left the Administration in disgust. These people have ranged all the way up to, and including, the Surgeon General of the United States. The Public Health Services hospital and clinic system has been of extreme interest to me over the years. For many individuals the system has been the primary and sometimes only source of health care. One of my main reasons for fighting so hard to keep these hospitals open is because they serve more than 400,000 merchant marines and countless other individuals who are in other services of the United States Armed Forces. They also have served as a very important secondary source for alternative health care to those communities that have health facilities that are being used to capacity or are already overloaded.

The closing of these hospitals would have a direct effect upon the economy of their surrounding areas, but even more important, the patients served by these hospitals would have nowhere to turn, unless of course they could bear the 40-50 percent higher cost of health care given in private hospitals.

The Administration has attempted to show that the closing of the hospitals will save some $35-45 million in renovation costs in the short run, but they fail to see that this initial saving would soon be consumed by the higher annual costs of providing care to merchant seamen and other PHS patients through community hospitals. Specifically, HEW's plans indicate that the proposal would cost about $8 million more each year than it now takes to keep the PHS hospitals going.

Even Dr. Wilson addressed this point:

The contention of the Administration that the closing of these hospitals would represent a cost saving for the federal government is deceptive. The cost of providing services to these beneficiaries through other means would be considerably greater than continuing care in the public health service hospitals.

It should also be kept in mind that the Public Health Service hospitals are more than buildings and facilities that serve patients. Each year Public Health Service hospitals train 12,000 physicians, dentists, medical technicians, licensed practical nurses, physician's assistants, orthopedic assistants, medical librarians, and other allied health personnel, in addition to the medical care they provide to well over one million Americans.

Dr. Wilson emphasized this point as well:

From a long range point of view, perhaps an even greater loss is the elimination of training programs. The hospitals have a rich tradition spanning more than two centuries of service and training. They constitute the main source of trained professionals for the public health service. Only the most naive could believe that a sufficient number of adequately trained public health professionals can be recruited from the acute care-oriented private sector. The cost of such recruitment and necessary additional training will be impressive.

135

The research programs of these hospitals are also important. The Public Health Service hospitals have had a long and enviable record of productive research, especially in such areas as cancer, hypertension, cardio-vascular disease, and other major killers. The bill that Congress passed and the President signed (Public Law 92-585) established conditions for the closing or transfer of Public Health Service facilities. The law required the Secretary of Health, Education and Welfare (HEW) to give detailed plans concerning any potential closing or transfers. No mention was made of the importance of the PHS contributions to research in the HEW-submitted proposal, and in fact, the reports did not even suggest that this kind of research should be continued.

It is difficult to overestimate the importance of Dr. Vernon Wilson's summary of the proposed hospital closings, especially since he was so intimately involved in the health programs of this Administration.

Dr. Wilson concluded:

> At a time when large numbers of citizens in the vicinities surrounding these eight hospitals are already inadequately served, it seems almost criminal to needlessly threaten the health or lose the lives of more citizens by destroying an uneconomically operated health care resource in the absence of viable alternatives for those whom it serves. Neither the population at large nor the government can afford to display such wanton disdain for life, health, and professional values.
>
> The time has come to take a responsible and publicly accountable look at the role of the federal government in direct health care, particularly through the Public Health Service. A blue ribbon citizen's group, supported by Congress, Executive Branch and health professionals at all levels, should study carefully the many proposals that are emanating from all branches of government. From such a study should develop a true plan, one which allows a constructive and dynamic transition from the present to the future. Perhaps the Public Health Service hospitals do need major changes.

If so, they should be instituted on a professionally sound basis. To do less denies all that we have been saying about the right of every citizen to health care.

The Public Health Service hospitals are not the only major facilities that have been under attack by the current Administration. When Administration health officials came to testify before our Senate Health Subcommittee on June 8, 1973, I zeroed in on the proposed elimination of the Medical Facilities Construction Act (Hill-Burton) and other regional medical programs. At this point, the Administration was represented by Dr. Frederick L. Stone, Acting Deputy Administrator for Development.

The first program examined was the Hill-Burton program. Most hospital bed construction for the last quarter century throughout this nation has been as a major consequence of the Hill-Burton program. Even the Administration has conceded the absolute success of this effort. Its argument is that because of the success of this program, and because we do not need an increase in hospital beds, Hill-Burton should be discontinued. But this is a fallacious and spurious conclusion.

It is true that on an overall basis there is not a need for greater numbers of hospital beds, but in several areas of this country, many of the existing hospital beds are outmoded, obsolete, and of highly questionable quality. Furthermore, Hill-Burton is no longer a program geared largely to providing additional hospital beds. In 1948, 80 percent of the funds went for additional beds, but last year the proportion was less than 5 percent. The overwhelming amount of dollars now goes for modernization programs, including public health centers, nursing home and chronic disease projects, outpatient facilities, and rehabilitation facilities.

There is no doubt that a need exists for modernization of facilities. Each state has a health planning agency that submits its professional estimate of present health facilities needs. For budget year 1974, The Department of Health, Education, and Welfare testified before Congress that states

137

indicated the need by 1980 of projects which would cost $2.4 billion dollars. At stake in the 1974 federal budget is whether approximately 350 health projects — and improved care for thousands of citizens — can be established.

With this in mind I asked Dr. Stone about the Hill-Burton program.

Dr. Stone: Medical facilities construction has assisted in the construction and modernization of public health and private non-profit hospitals and other health facilities through the Hill-Burton program. The program has been so singularly effective in improving the distribution of hospital beds to sections of the United States which were in short supply we were able to recommend that it be discontinued.

The other program scheduled to be phased out is the regional medical program (RMP). The major reason for the proposed termination of the RMP program is that it has not achieved its goal of getting medical advances rapidly into regular medical practice. The greatest expenditure of RMP funds has been in the area of continuing education and upgrading training of health personnel. The linkages which RMP was to establish between the research advantages of the categorial programs and the delivery of health care have not in fact been established.

I have been impressed by some of the fine RMP programs that I have been exposed to in the State of Washington. In the area of continuing education and upgrading of health personnel alone, the Washington/Alaska Regional Medical Program has trained nurse practitioners, established an education coordinator for eighteen small hospitals in North Central Washington and the Columbia Basin, trained nurses to staff coronary care units, and taught nurses to do electrocardiograms.

Some 16,000 Washington residents suffer stroke each

138

year. To help alleviate the situation, there must be adequate follow-up care and rehabilitation (particularly for people who live outside the metropolitan areas). Washington RMP has had to cut back on its program to train stroke nurses who would be able to provide competent therapy to the patient and counseling to the family. Reduced funding does not, of course, permit training enough nurses to meet the state's need.

Senator Magnuson: You say the greatest expenditure of the regional medical program funds has been in the area of continuing education, upgrading of health personnel. Don't you think that is important?

Dr. Stone: Yes, it is.

Senator Magnuson: How are you going to do it? How will you do it if you cut out all of the training and all of the other programs?

Dr. Stone: There are other programs.

Senator Magnuson: Why don't you say in RMP we ought to do more and make it better instead of saying just throw it out? Oh, well, you are not going to say it, so I am not going to belabor the point. I don't know why we hold these hearings, to be honest with you.

Mr. Miller: Mr. Chairman, question. (At this point, Mr. Charles Miller, Deputy Assistant Secretary overseeing the budget and a major Administration official sent to Capitol Hill to orchestrate the witnesses, attempted to interrupt).

Mr. Miller: Just two points. I want to set the record straight that we are not going to do something, just say to heck with what Congress is going to do, and we are just going to do it, because that is not so.

Mr. Miller was attempting to insert rationalizations and justifications on behalf of the Nixon Administration to explain why it has impounded funds for programs for which

139

Congress appropriated money. Again, the Administration missed the point of the hearings. The concern has to be with the impact these impoundments have upon the health of our citizens. Eliminating RMP would eliminate or force cutbacks in the Seattle Urban Indian Clinic, the training of emergency medical personnel in Pierce and Whatcom counties, and the Chicano Health Task Force — a group endeavoring to help Spanish-speaking people in the Northwest to find health care and to interest their young people in health-related careers.

Clearly such programs are important throughout the country, and should be kept and improved when necessary.

Senator Magnuson: Wait a minute, since when did this happen? Is this just coming along now?

Mr. Miller: We have not reached the point of final decision, Mr. Chairman.

Senator Magnuson: Oh, no, you make up your minds and that is it. And even if Congress does something, you just impound the funds. Now if you say we are going to have a better day, I am very pleased to hear that, but that hasn't been the experience.

I was still trying to get at who was making cutback recommendations within the Administration, and I kept trying. It was clear to all of us that the health professionals were really not for these program cutbacks.

Senator Magnuson: But the President or the Secretary doesn't make these recommendations unless somebody advises them down in your Department to do it.

Mr. Miller: Oh, sure.

Senator Magnuson: Now that is what I am trying to find out. Did Dr. Stone advise them to cut out the regional medical programs? Did you advise them to do that, Dr. Stone?

Dr. Stone: No, sir, it was a joint decision.

Senator Magnuson: Did you, yes or no?

Dr. Stone: No, sir, I did not.

140

Senator Stevens: (Senator Ted Stevens of Alaska is a
                     colleague on the Appropriations
                     Subcommittee. He is a Republican
                     Senator from Alaska and has also been
                     very active and critical of some of the
                     Administration's budget cuts in the health
                     areas.)
                     Mr. Miller. I hate to interrupt here but
                     you are doing it right now. We had an
                     agreement, we thought, in terms of the
                     continuing resolution, and we had a long
                     discussion here the other day about what
                     the continuing resolution means . . ., and
                     now here is the situation where you are
                     spending a lot less than you came up and
                     testified and supported in the budget last
                     year. We gave you the money that you
                     wanted, and you turned around and are
                     spending $214 million less in four
                     programs.
Mr. Miller: But, Senator, in between those occurrences you
                     had an absolute target in a total budget set
                     ($250 billion). Somehow, that had to be
                     reached. Now something had to give.
Senator Magnuson: Why did something have to give? We
                     passed the continuing resolution and
                     said "go ahead," and you people
                     interpreted it entirely different.
Mr. Miller: We did not have a viable appropriation that
                     could bring us to the $250 billion level.

Senator Stevens appeared shocked and chagrined to learn
that the Administration had impounded over $40 million in
the Hill-Burton appropriations. This was coupled with the
fact that Senator Aiken was being forced to introduce an
amendment to receive a half million dollars in Hill-Burton
funds for a much needed project in the State of Vermont.

Senator Stevens: Just a minute. We have an operating level

141

of $41.4 million and the Senator from Vermont, the ranking Republican on the floor of the Senate, asked to put in an amendment to get $500,000 authorized for Hill-Burton, and we are fighting in the supplemental budget trying to help Senator Aiken keep $500,000 when you have $41.4 million down there.

Mr. Miller: Yes, Senator, but. . .

Senator Magnuson: And that is just sitting there.

Senator Stevens: And you are not spending a dime of it, not a dime. You know, I agree with the Chairman. I don't know why sometimes we sit and listen because I don't know what you are going to do after I hear this.

You know you could at least spend at the 1972 budget year level. What you have done is cut out programs. You made an executive decision and cut out things without letting us know, and we have no control over it, according to you.

Suppose I put $41 million back there into Hill-Burton. Are you going to spend that?

Mr. Miller: I can't answer that.

Senator Magnuson: Why can't you? What is the purpose of us sitting here and holding hearings? If Congress decides that it wants $41 million in Hill-Burton and we hold all of these hearings, we can't get assurances you are going to spend it, anyway.

Mr. Miller: None at this table knows what we are going to spend.

Subsequent to these hearings, a number of interested groups in the health area have taken the Administration to court in order to have the funds released. In almost every instance, the judges have ruled against the Nixon Administration.

Senator Magnuson: What is the use of having these hearings, then?

Mr. Miller: This kind of dialogue is terribly critical because, Mr. Chairman, it is really not that much of a confrontation.

Senator Stevens: I'm telling you now that if you mislead us this time, I'm going to be out on the floor screaming that you really misled us also last year. It was this Department (HEW) that misled us. You did not tell us that you had a policy to do away with Hill-Burton. You did not tell us that you were going to do away with RMP capitation grants, nursing aid, and the rest of them, and you just did it, and now you are telling us we have decided the major reason for the proposed termination of RMP is that it has not achieved its goal.

You have already terminated it. It is misleading the Committee to say it was proposed because it was already done and you should come in and defend what you have done instead of telling us what you are going to do in the future.

Senator Magnuson: You came here last fall and told us to appropriate x-hundreds of millions of dollars for OEO. You said that was what you wanted. Two months later, you tell us that it was wrong, so Congress gets the blame for being the so-called big spender.

Senator Stevens: You know you heard me tee off before, but this is the worst one, because you haven't convinced the authorization committee to terminate RMPs, and as a matter of fact, their decision is just to the contrary.

So you are coming to us and saying, "Don't appropriate any more money for

143

RMPs" when the Congress has already made its determination and when the Senate Committee has already made its determination. So you people come right in here and say you are proposing to terminate RMP when you have hearings.

We've heard it now from the Secretary three times. We ask you questions that don't mean anything. You talk about something down the road that is going to happen and this and that, and you won't even wait until it happens. We have part of this bill which Mr. Miller knows depends upon special revenue sharing. You haven't even gotten special revenue sharing, and if this keeps up, I don't know if you are going to get any.

You say you don't make this decision, Dr. Stone?

Dr. Stone: I said it was a group decision.

Senator Magnuson: Well, what do you mean, were you in the group!

Dr. Stone: I was at my level of operation one of those.

Senator Magnuson: What group made the decision?

Dr. Stone: The ultimate decisions are made, I believe, in the OMB as a result of recommendations that come from above.

Senator Magnuson: All right. Why don't you come in and be honest and say the OMB cut us out? But we don't think they should cut us out of RMP, instead of coming in and saying we agree they should be cut out.

Do you agree they should be cut out?

Dr. Stone: I don't think it is an open and shut question, sir.

Senator Magnuson: You were in charge of this program, Dr. Stone.

Dr. Stone: Yes, sir.

Senator Magnuson: This is your shop, then. Nobody down at

the White House knows the details of this. They have to get some advice from you people. Now, did you advise them to close up all RMPs? Yes or no?

Dr. Stone: No, sir, I did not.

Senator Magnuson: All right, thank you very much. We will recess until Monday.

If you sense a certain anger and frustration in the above dialogue between Senator Stevens and myself and the Administration, there certainly was. On one hand, we were being told that a program like Hill-Burton was so successful that the Administration had no alternative but to phase it out, and on the other hand, the regional medical program had been such a failure that they had no alternative but to phase it out. In both cases, the Administration failed to reckon with the problems at hand, namely, whether or not the country has sufficient health facilities, and whether or not the latest advances in medicine are getting to the population at large. It is a shame that witnesses sent to the Hill by the Administration are often not allowed to give their honest professional opinion about programs such as these. And it is a shame that the pervading approach of the Nixon Administration has been to wrap their activities in a cloak of secrecy, and that this can even extend to programs for the physical well-being of our citizens.

Health facilities are not the only area in which the current Administration has attempted to cut back on the government's health commitment. Another has been medical manpower. Anyone who is even remotely familiar with health programs in the United States recognizes that we are in the midst of a shortage not only of trained and qualified doctors, but also of nurses, dentists, and other health professionals.

Some people have tried to propose that all we have is a maldistribution or overspecialization problem. That is merely semantics. The real problem is that citizens in this country who need medical care are not getting it, because they do not have access to a doctor. The example presented earlier in this book of Wolcott, Indiana describes the problem very well. There are many Wolcott, Indianas throughout the United States.

It is all too easy to point out several of these in the State of Washington. The Washington State Medical Education and Research Foundation located in Seattle did a study in 1970 of some aspects of the situation. The State of Washington presently has 5,400 physicians licensed to practice, or 161 for every 100,000 people. This ratio is slightly above the median for the country as a whole, and means that several states are significantly worse off than the State of Washington. But this figure itself is meaningless unless someone examines the spread throughout the state. It turns out that nearly two-thirds of the state's population live in the four most populous counties — Kings, Pierce, Snohomish, and Spokane. These counties have 78 percent of all of the physicians, indicating that other places in the state may be desperately in need of doctors. At latest count, the Medical Education and Research Foundation study indicated that seventy locations in the state were looking for doctors, particularly general practitioners. It is likely that the problem has gotten worse since that time.

This study also pinpointed areas that were in desperate need of physicians. For example, Forks, in Clallam County, with a population of 1,300, had only one GP who was contemplating retirement. The report suggested that Forks needed two GPs. North Bonneville in Skamania County, with a population of 452, had no physician but a doctor's office with equipment was available for reasonable rent. The nearest hospital was 29 miles east, in White Salmon. The entire county of 5,800 people had only one physician.

South Bend in Pacific County had a population of 1,720 with only one general practitioner, then aged 57, and a general surgeon, aged 58, along with a 39-bed general hospital. Since Pacific County had a population of 1,500, the two physicians in South Bend were attempting to serve an area with approximately 10,000 people. The Medical

146

Foundation estimated a need for two GPs immediately.

Sultan, in Snohomish County, had a population of over 1,100 with no physician and no hospital. Monroe, which is seven miles to the west, with a population of 2,700, had two physicians and a small hospital, but no physician or medical facility to the east, until far beyond the summit of the Cascade Pass. The report declared the need for a GP in Sultan immediately.

Connell, in Franklin County, had a population of 950. Because of the disability of the physician practicing in Connell, it was left doctorless. The Connell area is a trade center of over 3,500 people, and even has an excellent clinic building available.

These few examples should illustrate that there is indeed a manpower shortage, and that many areas not only in Washington but throughout the United States are either without or are short of doctors.

The Washington State Medical Education and Research Foundation concluded that Washington has a shortage of 936 general practice physicians. It is worthwhile to point out that Washington State is by no means atypical since, as stated before, it ranks slightly above the national average in the number of physicians per number of people in the state.

Startling needs such as these led me in 1970 to author a bill leading to the establishment of a National Health Service Corps. It was and still is clear that there is a physician shortage, and that the free market mechanism does not work to give the communities described above a chance to get general practicing doctors. This means that the only way to insure care for all of our citizens in these areas is to devise a government program to fill this void. Many people try to become fancy about the physician shortage and hide behind phrases like, "it's only a maldistribution problem, and what we really need is to have the doctors in overserved areas move out to underserved areas." Some people have an even fancier solution; they claim we have an over-supply of such things as neurosurgeons, and all we have to do is to have fewer surgeons and get more doctors to move out to areas like Wrangle, Alaska or Darrington, Washington (neither community having a physician).

The people who live in these towns without a doctor don't care whether the problem is a doctor shortage or a physician maldistribution or a preponderance of superspecialists. They are concerned that, when they need medical care, they can't get it. Anyway it is looked at, it spells not enough doctors providing services to people who need it.

The National Health Service Corps was created in order to improve and make available health services to those areas of urban and rural poverty where care is now inadequate. This Corps would be run under the Public Health Service in order to increase the quantity and quality of services in areas of the country that need them the most. We also wanted to provide a way for young health professionals and medical students to channel their idealism and social commitment toward helping and serving the most disadvantaged people in our nation.

I had occasion to visit Corpsmen in their practice in the State of Washington. One of the most exciting visits was to the Skamania County Hospital district in Stevenson, Washington. At that time, I had the privilege of meeting and talking with Dr. Rory M. Laughery, a young Corps physician.

I was extremely disturbed in November 1973 to receive a letter from Dr. Laughery indicating that the entire National Health Service Corps was in jeopardy.

Dr. Laughery cited two problems threatening the future of the Corps. The first related to making the salaries of NHSC competitive with those of MDs just starting out in practice. This problem is manageable through an upgraded pay scale that would be commensurate with that for physicians entering the Armed Services.

The second problem is pure and simple administrative bungling and bureaucratic molasses on the part of the HEW hierarchy. One very beneficial feature of the law creating the National Health Service Corps is its incentive to physicians who had been forced to borrow money to complete their physician training. The law called for such loans to be forgiven to those doctors agreeing to practice in critical health manpower shortage areas.

In October 1973, seventy young physicians learned that they would not get part of their medical education loans repaid because the bureaucrats in HEW were late in sending them the necessary forms. The forms had not been sent until June 15, 1973, or nineteen months after the manpower acts were passed and eight months after clarifying amendments were added through the passage of federal legislation. This made it impossible for new physicians scheduled to begin their tour of service on July 1, 1973 to return the agreement contracts. Word of this has filtered through to medical schools and medical centers across the country where the Corps has to recruit future members, and can have nothing short of disastrous consequences.

Many have accused the Nixon Administration of intentionally trying to subvert this program, and trying again to circumvent laws that Congress has passed.

I would like to feel that this is not true, and that it was just a bureaucratic foul-up. In any case, it will make getting health care in Forks, North Bonneville, South Bend, Sultan and Connell much more difficult in 1975 than it was in 1973. If most people believe, as I do, that the federal government has a responsibility to make sure that doctors are available in communities like this throughout the country, then the President must be made aware of it.

The role of government here is to provide incentives, and hope that the medical community, including medical students, medical schools and organized medicine, will make such a program work. The National Health Service Corps is still in an experimental phase. I look forward to it becoming permanent.

On June 5, 1974, along with Senators Edward Kennedy and Jacob Javits I introduced a proposal to extend the Corps for another five years. The NHSC represents the first major step to directly confront the maldistribution of health care personnel, and while mandating national service for health graduates may not be the best solution, it is an approach that is certainly worth close scrutiny.

I am proud of the active role I played in the creation of the Corps, and hope very much that it will work, because frankly, the alternatives to meeting the national health manpower crisis are not as easy to face.

Dr. H. McDonald Rimple, while Director of the National Health Service Corps, described its creation as "one of the great humanitarian challenges of this decade." In describing the program, Dr. Rimple commented:

> The Act authorizes the Corps to place health teams consisting of physicians, dentists and allied health professionals in areas of critical health manpower shortage. In many of these shortage areas, the physician/population ratio is greater than 1 to 5,000. In many of our counties, there are no physicians at all.
>
> Basically what we are doing is helping communities to help themselves. In our brief experience of providing medical and dental assistance to rural and urban areas which had been without it, we have encountered heartening models of communities organizing their resources and ingenuity to share with us in the delivery of quality health care.

In describing the National Health Service Corps, a Public Health Service publication indicated that:

> Corpsmen are where the action is, dealing with people, making hard and fast decisions, fighting to solve life and death problems.

This report also gave many examples of the fine cooperation that developed between communities and Corps members, such as two Corps physicians serving residence in an urban renewal area in Decatur, Georgia, a suburb of Atlanta. Their clinic is a renovated apartment in the Kirkwood housing complex. Before the Corps physicians arrived, Kirkwood residents were served by only one physician. Today, the Corps team is building a solid practice

150

with excellent support from the local medical society. Both doctors have admitting privileges at DeKalb General Hospital.

The National Health Service Corps includes not only trained doctors, but also dentists, nurses, and other health professionals. It has been virtually impossible for poor communities to attract and retain sufficient health professionals to meet even their most basic health needs. The consequences of this inadequate health care are physically, socially, and economically crippling to the poorer citizens, and shameful for our nation as a whole.

Some health problems that are routine and even trivial in the richer communities become serious and near fatal in those areas where access to health care is severely restricted. The diseases of poverty, including higher infant mortality rates, shorter life expectancies, malnutrition, anemia, and so on become worse when untreated, and they contribute substantially to reinforcing the circle of poverty and low economic productivity.

When I introduced the National Health Service Corps concept, I knew that it would not eliminate all of these diseases, nor would it solve completely the problems that we have in providing sufficient health manpower. However, it will help in providing incentives for young physicians to serve, at least for a few years, in areas that desperately need health care.

10.   Health Care Delivery

"What's Wrong With American Medicine?" asked a headline in the *Reader's Digest* of April 1973. Author Donald C. Drake answered that:

> ... too many people can't get adequate care and too many others can't afford it when it is available. But now the whole system is on the threshold of major change.

The story described:

> ... an old man (who) walked into the municipal hospital of one of the nation's largest cities recently and asked the registration clerk if he could see a doctor. Told to wait, the old man obediently took a seat at the back of the crowded room. An hour later ... he died — a fact not discovered until hours later.

Other examples included:

> Mrs. Susan Bonnell of Philadelphia, (who) unlike the old man, didn't have to depend on a deteriorating city hospital for medical care. Because she was covered by medical insurance, she could pick any hospital she wanted when she was stricken last year by a kidney infection that hospitalized her six times. Mistakenly believing that her insurance would pay the bills, she was shocked when she learned that she had used up her allotment of covered days and owed a hospital bill of about $3,000.

Mrs. Mary Wilt of Dover, Delaware, mother of seven girls, and her husband, a warehouseman, can't afford private medical care. "Every time you go to the clinic you get a different doctor," she reports. "You never get a chance to get to know a face or gain confidence in one doctor. Because you get state aid, you can just feel that I-don't-care-about-you attitude."

Under our present health-care system, too many Mrs. Wilts are being demeaned, too many Mrs. Bonnells being bankrupted and too many old men dying unnoticed.

In contrast, the following case was presented by Natalie Spingarn, a freelance health writer.

Seattle, Washington. On a July day three years ago, Leif E. Grefsrud was working by lamplight on his car in the garage of his home nineteen miles south of here. Suddenly, gasoline began pouring out of the auto.

The 36-year old Boeing engineer, fearful of fire, crawled out from under the car, and pulled out the lamp plug. There was a spark, and the gasoline burst into flames — as did Grefsrud, who ran outside screaming. A neighbor ran to turn a hose on him while Grefsrud rolled in the grass in agony. 75 percent of his body ended up covered with burns, one-half of them third degree.

After a few days at a nearby hospital, to which he had been rushed, Grefsrud was moved to the hospital of Group Health Cooperative of Puget Sound, where he underwent six months of intensive and extensive care: special nurses round-the-clock for two and one-half months, surgeons performing eight skin grafts, in addition to his regular doctor's treatment, specialists providing physical therapy, laboratory work, drugs, intravenous feedings. After leaving the hospital six months later, Grefsrud had to return at least half a dozen times for plastic surgery on his fingers, arms, and ears.

The normal cost of all this care is estimated at $25,000.

The cost to Grefsrud: $40 a month at first, $50 a month later, and that included medical coverage for his wife and three children as well.

The kind of care provided this family is called pre-paid, and is provided through the growing body of clinics called health maintenance organizations, or HMOs.

Until the last few years — except for a small number of people mostly on the east or west coasts — most medical care has been obtained by the fee for service method, or going to a doctor when sick and paying a given fee. This method of paying for medical care has been the choice of the bulk of the American population, but it is not the only way, or necessarily the right way, for every family. It is equally true that although the number of HMOs has been increasing at a slow pace over the last few years, they may not be the best choice for every family.

However, it is a healthy sign that HMOs are becoming available in enough places in this country that some families can decide which approach is best for their particular needs. It is essential for health consumers to be aware of how their health dollar gets spent, and what alternatives they have. The recent passage of an HMO bill (December 1973) by Congress indicated for the first time government's concern with the organization and delivery of health services to the public.

It is of interest to look at the Group Health Cooperative of Puget Sound as an example of an HMO. It has some unique features which cannot be replicated in other places, but might serve as a useful example of lessons we can learn. Also, it has stood the test of time. Originally organized in 1944, it now faces the problem that too many people want to enroll in the plan. Finally, the major reason for looking at this plan is that it is a consumer-owned cooperative.

Group Health was originally formed by some 200 members of the Grange, the Aero-Mechanics Union, and other Seattle residents. They decided to organize around four basic principles: (1) control of the cooperative would rest with the members rather than doctors (2) the election of trustees and major policy decisions would be made on a one-member, one-vote basis (3) so far as possible, a single monthly payment would cover all the health care costs of member families and (4) emphasis would be placed on health education and preventive medicine.

Group Health's path has not always been smooth. For example, in 1953, the entire Cooperative almost collapsed when consumer trustees reinstated a doctor that the medical staff had fired. But out of that bitter dispute emerged a new Joint Conference Committee, consisting of three doctors and three trustees, to which all potential conflicts between consumers and medical staff have since been referred. Now, twenty years later, Group Health Cooperative has approximately 180,000 members, and new enrollment has had to be restricted.

One major reason for this movement to medical cooperatives is probably the disappearance of the general practitioner. Dr. Alex Gerber, in *The Gerber Report,* described how Americans:

> . . . remember the old-time general practitioner out of a Norman Rockwell painting: driving far out to a lonely farmhouse in the middle of the night to deliver a baby, wiping the brow of a feverish child, or draining pus from the chest by lamplight on the kitchen table (in how many movies did you see the doctor take off his coat, roll up his sleeves with determination and say, "Get me hot water — lots of hot water"! The doctor was family counselor and friend, ministering angel and miracle worker all rolled into one.

Dr. Gerber then goes on to describe how the general practitioner could fit the health needs of the future:

> The direction of training and practice has shifted heavily toward specialization, not only in the United States, but all over the world. In 1931, GPs outnumbered specialists five to one. Now, this ratio is almost completely reversed. Physicians in general practice comprise less than 20 percent of the total physician population, and 18 percent

of them are over 65 years of age. Specialists, on the other hand, rose from 14,000 in 1939 to 112,000 in 1970.

Over time, medicine has moved more and more to group practice, which offer advantages both to doctors and patients. Just as the term "HMO" is getting bandied about, so the term "group practice" means many different things to many people. To some, it is the sharing of common facilities by two or more physicians where each continues to handle his own kind of organization and his own patients. They may share a secretary or perhaps equipment such as the x-ray machine.

A more formal arrangement is when physicians band together to form a partnership. They not only share expenses and facilities, but also pool their income and divide it according to some prearranged plan. There are really two different kinds of group practices. In one, all of the physicians in the practice have the same specialty, for example, all obstetricians or pediatricians. The other kind of group practice may include doctors in many specialties, such as internists, pediatricians, obstetricians, and possibly even a surgeon.

Multi-specialty groups have the advantage of providing the consumer with a chance to get all his care in one spot, much as in the supermarket, which has now taken the place of a number of small grocery and variety shops.

When physicians are asked why they go into groups, they give a number of reasons, such as the chance to have more free time, equipment and personnel which they could probably not afford if they practiced alone; and accident and sickness benefits, more reasonable insurance rates, and retirement plans generally unavailable to lone practitioners. From the standpoint of care, if a patient has a particularly puzzling illness, there is an opportunity to consult with other members of the team if they are located nearby.

The most important aspect of multi-specialty group practices is that they can provide comprehensive care. Over the years, in constituents' complaints to me about the health care system, the item that is always close to the top of the list is the depersonalized fragmentation of service. People are left to figure out how to handle too many care decisions by themselves. My constituents convinced me long ago that we should do whatever possible to provide consumers with more personalized and comprehensive care, both in terms of how that care is delivered and how we pay for it.

In October 1973, *Medical Economics* assembled 110 handpicked health experts to predict medical changes over the next five years. Their overwhelming consensus was that the public was looking for an increase in the "art" of medicine, in other words greater personalized care by health practitioners.

It has only been recently, however, that people have felt their care system could be changed. They have begun to look toward government for some rationale for the medical care and health care system. This is certainly not true of organized medicine, but even the American Medical Association has mellowed over time, as evidenced by their active participation in the establishment of Professional Standards Review Organizations (PSROs), mentioned before as a new federal program to assess and insure that quality care is provided to health consumers. In many ways, this program is a partnership between the public and the doctors, who have indicated that they would like an opportunity to police themselves in cutting abuses and overuses and overprescriptions by their fellow practitioners.

It is important for the public to know that one intention of recent federal legislation is to provide a better health care system. The government should not step in and run or even manage hospitals or nursing homes or other health care facilities, but should act, as in the establishment of the National Health Service Corps, on the assumpton that it is the proper role of the federal government to stimulate use of our resources to bring care to people who need it.

It was with this philosophy in mind that a number of us co-sponsored legislation leading to the passage of the Health Maintenance Organization (HMO) Act of 1973.

It should be pointed out again that even the most

exuberant HMO advocates have never claimed that HMOs could or should be for everyone. In fact, many experts and a number of recent polls and questionnaires have concluded that no more than 20-25 percent of the people in this country would join such plan. But approximately 8 million people do belong to such plans, and another 35 or 40 million Americans would probably want the opportunity to participate in such a program.

The first and most successful consumer-based HMO was the Group Health Cooperative of Puget Sound. The officials at Group Health believe that the success and the quality of health care which they provide is due primarily to the major involvement of their members and their unique consumer-provider-manager team. While Congress was considering action on the HMO legislation, the Board of Trustees of Group Health offered basic concepts in testimony to the Senate which they believed should be used by organizations providing health care. First and foremost was the suggestion of maximum consumer involvement and consumer rights:

> The rise of the consumer movement indicates clearly a desire for accountability of institutions supported by tax funds to the citizens these institutions are intended to serve. In other words, consumers are not satisfied anymore to have federal agencies charged with the responsibility of implementation of laws. Experience at Group Health during the past twenty-five years shows ever increasing benefits to its subscribers by the utilization of consumers who are experts in a number of fields involved in health care delivery.

In effect, members who receive health care volunteer some of their special talents. These consumers of health encompass a wide range of occupations such as businessmen, architects, lawyers, builders, and finance and management leaders. Their experience and creative ideas help the health professional solve some of the complex problems presented by modern health care delivery.

159

As Group Health describes it, the participation and accountability of consumers has resulted in the following benefits:

—An increase in responsiveness to consumer needs, and hence in the quality of health delivery as the consumer perceives it.

—A creative partnership between consumers and providers resulting in a community of interest and an identification of the consumer with his organization. The consumer becomes an active participant.

—A constant flow of new ideas from consumers who seek change to provide better benefits and services.

—An effective means of quality and cost review.

—A sharing of savings. Consumers will be able to share in financial savings generated by the program and help support it vigorously.

This adds up to allowing the consumers more say about how the plan takes shape, and builds in incentives to make the program more efficient. When this happens, the savings are not in the form of profits to some big company, but rather the benefits return to the people participating in the program.

People who belong to Group Health fall generally into one of two categories. The first is the individual "co-op member" and his family. This group comprises almost 40 percent of all the enrollees. The co-op member enrolled on an individual family basis pays an initial capital investment in the form of an interest-free loan of $175, plus $25 for initial processing and health examination. After that, the monthly dues for a co-op family of four are about $48, and that includes comprehensive health care coverage, including prescription drugs.

Almost 60 percent of the members joined through their group contract at their place of employment, generally an industrial-labor or a government worker's contract. There are over 15,000 federal employees who participate in Group Health. The monthly dues for a family of four under this plan are also close to $50. HEW has estimated that the basic services under the HMO legislation will be $70-$75 per month, which if true may make it difficult for new HMOs to compete. It is interesting to note that the costs per year for a family of four will be something like $600 at Group Health, which should be compared with the national average of health expenses for every person in this country, which comes to $440 per person annually, or $1,760 for a family of four.

It might be worthwhile for a family to compare a year's potential health expenses in belonging to an HMO to average costs for a year not covered by such a plan. The health care contracts with Group Health includes lifetime coverage as well as medical and surgical care in home, outpatient clinic, or hospital, as well as preventive health measures, x-rays, laboratory services, and physical therapy when needed. It includes nearly all prescription drugs, medications and surgical supplies, private duty nurses and other service as ordered by doctors, and offers mental health care with ten visits without charge and $5.00 per visit thereafter.

A consumer may have as many doctor visits for medical treatment and diagnosis as needed. Pediatric care, including baby checkups and immunizations, and costs for x-rays and other kinds of laboratory tests, eye examinations, and emergency care are all covered under this kind of a program.

The advocates of Group Health feel that owning their own hospital, controlling the hospital's policies, having a voice in its management, and relating all these activities to their outpatient services is what keeps their efficiency at such a high level. In addition, they feel that their costs are lower than for other methods of delivering health care.

One of the ways in which Group Health has studied cost differences is through the nearly 8,000 memebers that they have enrolled under contracts covering the Model Cities and welfare families in King County. Dr. H. Frank Newman, Director and Chief Administrator of the program, described some of the details on cost when he appeared before the Senate Committee on Finance looking into health care in April 1971. According to Dr. Newman, the care of low income groups costs the government two-thirds of the money

161

government must spend in caring for welfare families not under Group Health coverage. In other words, if the federal government went out to buy the same package of services from someone other than Group Health, the price would be 50 percent higher.

Another standard of comparison is the number of days spent in the hospital. It turns out that people using Group Health, and this also seems true for other pre-paid group practice plans, require hospitalization only about one-half to two-thirds as much as those who receive care on a fee for service basis. There seem to be a number of factors involved.

A study done for the February 1971 issue of the Harvard *Law Review* indicated that, in general, the major savings from hospitalization were correlated with a lower rate of surgery. The study found that those who were in pre-paid group practice plans had half as many appendectomies as those in the fee for service system. They had one-fourth as many tonsillectomies and adenoidectomies, and half as many female surgeries. This kind of measurement is very important, particularly when a noted surgeon like Alex Gerber indicates that there are more surgical operations in this country than necessary. Even more startling is the estimate by Dr. Denenberg, former Insurance Commissioner of the State of Pennsylvania, that there are as many as two million unnecessary surgeries each year in the United States.

A December 1973 editorial in the *New England Journal of Medicine* indicated that too many surgeries may be harmful. This editorial reported a study suggesting "some of the excess mortality (this was a study of gall bladder operations) may conceivably be attributed to the increased surgery." The article, written by Dr. John Bunker and Dr. John Wennberg (of Harvard Medical School) holds that:

> there is evidence that rates for some other operations may exceed their therapeutic usefulness — that operations designed to decrease death may, when performed in excess, increase it.

Obviously, if scientific evidence shows that extra

operations not only line the pockets of greedy doctors but also are harmful to the public, this practice must be ended.

Another area in which Group Health cuts costs is in having its own hospital, which because it is owned by the consumers who also have to pay the bills, carries a built-in incentive to limit unnecessary and expensive surgery and avoid a surplus of beds and equipment.

Proponents of pre-paid plans argue that their system focuses more on preventive health care, in the long run reducing the need for expensive surgery, while tending to catch many illnesses at a much earlier stage. They argue that early doctor and clinic visits are preventive health measures and turn out to be a much less costly and more humane way to provide medical care. The pre-paid philosophy is that proper and complete outpatient care reduces the need for hospital care to a low but appropriate level.

When one compares the Group Health statistics with the national average, it is evident that people enrolled in Group Health have many more doctor's visits than the national average. In fact, there are five visits to doctors for every four by the general population. On the other hand, the most expensive kind of care, namely care within hospitals, is much lower than the national average. Under Group Health, ninety people for every 1,000 belonging to the plan would enter the hospital in a given year, compared to the national average of 140 people out of every 1,000. Under Group Health, the length of a person's hospital stay is less than five days, whereas the national average is 8.3 days.

The total annual cost of care to someone who belonged to Group Health in 1970 was $143 for every person, compared with $226 for similar services to an average person not enrolled in such a plan.

The governing board of the cooperative is elected from and by the membership. This board meets at least each month, sets the policy, studies and analyzes problems, and conducts business for the cooperative. There are also about a dozen subcommittees which serve the board and are composed of members of the medical staff and the cooperative. These committees meet monthly to investigate the matters assigned to them by the board and make recommendations. There are also eight district organizations that meet quarterly for discussion and review of the board and committee actions, and for health education programs.

A major feature of the cooperative is a complaint department, where a patient who has something to say about the care can register his comments and suggestions. Last year, this program handled 9,000 "patient contacts". This means that out of every 15 enrollees, one availed himself of the service, usually to request information, as well as voice complaints. There is also a counselling program with a 24-hour-a-day phone system run by two nurse consultants. If the nurse consultant feels she can't handle the complaint by phone, she can reach one of the doctors on duty in the emergency department, or the patient's own doctor. Questions received are usually requests for information. About 1,300 of the complaints were about overcrowded facilities, including inadequate parking. There were about 300 complaints about the kind of medical care given, and these ranged from arranging appointments to complaints about service or attitudes, and 56 complaints about physicians.

These complaints are taken up with the medical section and area chiefs. When there are too many against one doctor, they show up in the strict system of peer review, under which the doctors periodically evaluate each other's performance.

Group Health Cooperative of Puget Sound seems to be living proof that consumers can organize to promote and protect public health and operate most effectively in their own best interests. This kind of organization grew from ordinary people out of shops, offices and kitchens, all interested in receiving comprehensive quality health care.

As one of its sponsors I was delighted by the passage of the original Health Maintenance Organization legislation written by Senator Edward Kennedy of Massachusetts. This bill is a first step by the federal government in coming to grips with the fragmentation of organization in the health care industry. Some of the important consumer protection features of the Group Health Cooperative of Puget Sound were incorporated in the final provisions of this bill. To me, another important aspect was the federal government's recognition that (just as the government had to step in to protect our elderly citizens because of exorbitant health care costs in the enactment of Medicare) we must also be concerned about the organization and accessibility of health care to the public at large. The bill also required the government to be concerned about the quality of health care delivered. An added feature is a stipulation that the average worker have a choice of an HMO as well as the more traditional employee health benefit package that he is normally offered.

In many ways, this legislation will provide a more diversified and competitive approach to delivering health care. Few people would argue that HMOs are for everyone, but it is clear to me, now that Group Health in Seattle cannot accommodate all who would like to join, that somewhat more than the 3-4 percent of Americans now enrolled in HMOs would like to do so, and that this Act will make it easier for them.

One of the greatest successes of the Group Health Cooperative program is the power and control that is wielded by the average cooperative member. It is with particular pleasure that I note the expanded role for the consumer under these new health maintenance organizations. The Secretary of Health, Education and Welfare will be required to assess the care given in these programs, and our highly important health delivery system must now under Federal law be looked at from the consumer's standpoint. Unfortunately, the tugs and pulls of the legislative process produced a bill of much more limited scale than is currently needed. But the important principle of government responsibility has been established, with the essential recognition that health care is too important to be left to doctors alone, and that other health care providers, as well as the consumers of these services, should have a voice in this decision-making.

11. Health Financing

CASE NUMBER ONE:
A sixty-two year old man (Mr. P.) developed heart trouble and had to retire. He drew $81 a month Social Security and could not afford medical insurance. When he had to enter the hospital, a $400 deposit was required. His daughter and her husband paid it out of the $700 they had saved over a fourteen year period, and his son paid the rest of the $2,000 hospital bill. Then he was diagnosed as having lung cancer. His daughter's husband, Larry, writes: "We have been to Social Security and they say they can do nothing. We went to welfare; they said that Medicaid does not cover him. We pay taxes and we stand for Medicaid and then it doesn't cover it. The children he had have spend all their money; the old man has spent all of his money. What are we going to do now? We can't just let him die."

It seems to me that when a man has worked for fifty years and paid taxes, he ought to be able to rest and take life easy without having to worry about having enough money to pay some hospital or doctor.

This case and the others included below were submitted to the Senate by the AFL-CIO Department of Community Services in October 1971. They are typical of several hundred others presented.

CASE NUMBER TWO:
A twenty-one year old man faced bankruptcy because of medical expenses incurred when his wife had a baby. He

was discharged from the Navy a short while before the baby was born, and thought that his service insurance would cover the birth. A new law made this impossible, leaving the couple with a large hospital bill and two good-sized doctors' bills. The husband was underemployed, making just enough to put him above the income standards set up by public welfare agencies and was also faced with expensive surgery for the removal of a growth from his ear not be covered by insurance because he had not had his policy long enough.

This case is a good example of a number of gaps and loopholes in our health care system. When in the armed forces, this young man was protected, but now that he is trying to get started on the right foot with a new youngster at home, he must either run into debt, or forego needed ear surgery, or go on public assistance to protect himself and his family. Is it any wonder that there is a hue and cry for national health insurance from many quarters today?

CASE NUMBER THREE:

A fifty-four year old Wisconsin woman had to quit work because of arteriosclerosis. Her group insurance wouldn't accept her and because she was not totally disabled, she didn't qualify for Social Security disability benefits. Too young for Medicare, she asked: "What can a person in my predicament do except urge Congress to pass a bill for universal health insurance?"

CASE NUMBER FOUR:

The wife of a textile worker was hospitalized for two weeks due to a miscarriage with complications. The hospital bill was $1,994, of which the insurance paid $1,299. The worker owed the balance of $695. He was eligible for Medicaid and received payment for one week. The insurance company took so long to make their payment that the time limitation for public assistance expired and Medicaid would not pay the $425 remaining.

These examples vividly demonstrate the absurdities that

pervade our present health care system. The consequences are disastrous. People striken with a serious illness not only risk losing their jobs but also risk losing the health insurance provided by their employer when they need the coverage the most.

Getting caught "between the cracks" and back and forth in the bureaucratic maze happens much too often. I have been a constant critic of the extraordinary bureaucracy that has developed around payment for health care, both in government programs such as Medicaid and in the screening procedures of private insurance companies. Sometimes, as in the case of the textile worker's wife, the maze becomes so circular that no one pays and the consumer faces disaster.

These cases are not even among the worst as far as large bills are concerned, and in fact many of these individuals can consider themselves lucky to be getting proper care. The worst cases are those in which people who need care can't find the practitioners who will provide it, and couldn't pay for it if they did.

Americans should not be turned down for care because they do not have the money. Yet with costs rising as fast as they are and with the gaps in insurance coverage, this will become more of a problem for more consumers.

The National Consumer Information Center (NCIC) predicts that the cost of medical care in the United States by 1975 will be double what it was in 1968:

Because the potential cost of serious illness is so great, the purchase of health insurance is especially important for the consumer. The 1970 statistics show that, while 80 percent of the American population has some form of health insurance, only 30 percent of the public's medical bills were paid by the insurance industry, which only goes to illustrate the need for careful planning in the purchase of health insurance. The consumer should be aware of what coverage is available through private and government plans, analyze his or her needs, and then decide on a health insurance package which best suits his or her needs.

169

Health insurance operates on the principle of spreading the risk among those who have insurance. But in practice this has not worked well, and people who get sick often find that there are large gaps and deficiencies in their insurance policies.

An example of a good insurance program is Medicare, which covers senior citizens through Social Security. This is a fair way to spread the costs among the elderly as well as Social Security payers in general. If it did not exist, those who got sick would have all of their assets wiped out in no time at all. However, even the Medicare program has serious deficiencies. As was pointed out earlier, high inflation has worked to cut back benefits, and there have even been cases of a few doctors taking unfair advantage of the program. These factors cause elderly citizens to pay more money out of their own pockets now than when the program began.

The February 1974 Nixon health plan further erodes care for elderly citizens. While a small percentage will fare better financially, the vast majority will be hurt by this new proposal. The National Council of Senior Citizens has indicated that under the Nixon plan ". . . 95 percent of the elderly will not be helped, and out-of-pocket costs will soar." Today's average hospital bill to the senior citizen of $84 will rise to $342. A thirty day stay will be nine times as costly, from today's $84 to $750.

In 1973, $132 for health care was paid out-of-pocket for every man, woman, and child in this country. This is over and above the amount of money paid for by government or insurance, whether it be private insurance or Blue Cross. The total amount of money spent for health care in 1973 averaged $441 for every man, woman, and child. There is no better example of the problems encountered in out-of-pocket expenses than Case Number One at the beginning of this chapter, in which Mr. P. and his children were left with no way to pay for his illness.

The paying of health cost bills must be made more equitable from a financial standpoint, and it is appropriate for the federal government to serve as standard-setter and protector. It should not be necessary for the government either to provide the care or pay for it all. Insurance payments can come from employers as well as employees and should allow for incentives to provide the broadest possible coverage. For example, if it is possible for insurance companies to protect the consumer while not making exorbitant profits, this should be explored. However, the large state by state differences in benefits existing under Medicaid should be discouraged. Proposals that are based on means to pay and are long on deductibles and short on benefits turn out merely to shortchange the consumer.

Americans spent $94 billion on health care in fiscal 1973 and will spend $104 billion in fiscal 1974. The current system is inequitable and will bankrupt many and cause thousands of others to go without care because of the expense and thereby become disabled or die. This situation must be changed.

For those of us who believe that medical care should be available to everyone in this nation as a fundamental right and not a privilege for those able to afford it, the question of health insurance is of utmost importance. Professor I. S. Falk, Professor Emeritus of Public Health at the Yale School of Medicine, summed it up this way:

> Because availability of medical care has become in larger and larger measure a matter of cost, the two threads — the concern for availability and the need for cost-sharing — have become permanently intertwined and the issue of national health insurance is the culmination of these originally severable concerns.

I have been convinced by hundreds upon hundreds of witnesses before the Senate over the years that the two areas the public most fears financially are automobile accidents and health problems. That is why the federal government should provide the proper setting and standards for all citizens to have comprehensive automobile and health insurance in order to protect against such catastrophic economic wipe-outs.

There has been some progress in health insurance over the past several years but much more needs to be done. Prog-

171

ress to date has been due to the inclusion of health provisions in management-union contracts to cover all or part of the medical costs of employed individuals. Some group coverage for health care has also been extended to a larger segment of the population.

In addition to private health insurance programs, nearly all of our elderly population is now covered through the national Medicare program, and many of the poor and near-poor have a corresponding group payment through the federal-state programs known as Medicaid. Progress in all of these areas has certainly been positive, and the insurance industry now points with pride to the close to 180 million persons who have "some form" of health insurance protection. In many cases, however, the "form" is lacking a great deal of substance.

A picture very different from the one painted by the insurance industry emerges when the individual consumer or family is considered. In budget year 1973, Americans spent $94 billion for personal health services. Of that amount, all forms of government (federal, state and local) provided 40 percent or $37.6 billion. Of the remaining $56.5 billion, private insurance covered approximately $20 billion, and approximately $28 billion was paid by the individual consumer out of his or her pocket. This area of expenditures by average citizens should be closely examined. Many of these expenditures are small and easily manageable, and include individual visits to doctors for minor colds or drugs, eyeglasses, or other kinds of relatively inexpensive forms of care.

But also included in that $94 billion sum are the very expensive, burdensome and sometimes catastrophic illnesses that can wipe out a family's total income and all of their savings. For 25 million Americans, the situation is acute — they are uninsured, need insurance the most, and are least able to obtain it. But disaster can also strike those families who think they have private, comprehensive health insurance. After a major illness or accident hits, they often find out how very limited and inadequate their health insurance is. It is because no individual or family can know for sure whether they will have large-scale medical expenses that comprehensive health insurance is such an important requirement.

Rapidly escalating medical costs have reached a crisis stage. In 1930, personal health service expenditures were $3.3 billion, whereas in 1970 they reached $60 billion, and in 1974 will exceed $100 billion. Part of this increase, of course, is due to the rise in population. But while population doubled between 1930 and 1970, medical costs went up seventeenfold in that period, so that the price of health per individual was eight and one-half times what it was in 1930. High costs continued on a runaway course, in spite of stringent requirements under the Economic Stabilization Act.

Americans must not be fooled by artificial or partial price tags placed on new health insurance proposals. For example, many experts have indicated that the 1974 Nixon Administration insurance proposal would cost the government treasury less than the Health Security proposal. On the basis of direct costs this is probably true, but that tells only a part of the story.

The point is that the total cost of health care to the consumer will be the same under either plan — close to $100 billion in 1974, $111 billion in 1975, and over $120 billion in 1976. The consumer will bear these costs either exclusively or in combination by paying for an expansion of the Social Security program, by paying private health insurance premiums, or by paying directly out of his pocket. It should be noted that no matter what approach is chosen the government will not be telling doctors how to practice medicine.

The Nixon Administration proposal would require the average American family to pay between one-third to one-half of an average $625 annual insurance premium. Hence, $200 to $300 would come out of a consumer's pocket — for premium payments and would only provide partial coverage. In addition, families would pay up to $1,500 out-of-pocket for illnesses because of a complicated series of deductibles. The Administration plan would cost consumers at least $12.4 billion in out-of-pocket expenses just for doctors and hospitals. Overall, the Nixon plan would cost consumers an estimated $29 billion out-of-pocket while the health security program would cost consumers $18 billion in out-of-pocket expenses.

The other major difference between the two approaches is that the Nixon Plan would raise $42 billion by requiring employers and employees to purchase private insurance, while the health security program would provide for similar payment through the tried and proven Social Security program. An important consideration is that at least $6 billion of the $42 billion private insurance costs is estimated to go to company profits and not to health care.

There is nothing wrong with private insurance companies administering national health insurance, but not at the expense of the consumer. National standards and criteria must make sure that the health consumer comes first and cost escalation slows down.

Dr. I. S. Falk has analyzed many of these cost considerations in historical perspective:

During the past two decades, the nation has become first concerned and then outraged by the continuing escalation of medical care costs at a pace much faster than the prices generally and faster than the rapid growth of the national economy. After 1965, a consensus began to emerge to the effect that the difficulty over cost and payment did not stand alone and could not be dealt with alone. Despite higher and higher costs, charges and payments, public as well as private, medical care was become increasingly difficult to obtain and large areas and population groups were seriously underserved. Comprehensiveness of services was not being achieved, despite the enlarging of expenditures. Quality of care was getting no better for many people, despite widely publicized expansion of medical knowledge, and

174

achievements of promising new medical skills. The institutions responsible for professional and technical training of the health manpower needed for a growing population and for the expanding demand for health services were in progressively deepening fiscal straits. The whole medical care system — or "non-system" as many began to call it — was in trouble and needed an overhauling.

It is for precisely these reasons that the public has begun to demand that the federal government take a stronger hand in the development of a rational health system. This demand by the public has led to the series of new health initiatives undertaken by the Congress in the past few years. The progressive steps have been by and large incremental. This is all the more reason for a national policy to provide health care when needed, and to require simultaneous improvement and development of resources for care along with a manageable and equitable way of paying for it.

Over the years, a number of proposals for a national health insurance policy have been made. In fact, in 1949, a landmark proposal was introduced by Senators Thomas, Murray, Wagner, Humphrey and Pepper for a "program of national health insurance and public health . . . to assist in increasing the number of adequately trained professional and other health personnel." I was pleased to be a sponsor of that far-reaching proposal. Unfortunately, this strong initiative twenty-five years ago under President Truman was ahead of its time.

I am happy to note that many aspects of that proposed legislation have been implemented in more recent times. In looking back I sometimes regret that the climate at that time prevented the passage of our original national health program. The strong emphasis on research and prevention for children would be paying back great dividends today.

The Truman Administration, following the unsuccessful health initiatives of 1949, proposed a program in 1951 that would have insured seven million Social Security beneficiaries for sixty days of hospital care. That proposal became the forerunner of the Medicare program.

The enactment of Medicare and Medicaid in 1965 with strong support by President Lyndon Johnson was a giant step forward in protecting a portion of the population against medical costs. Since then, however, there have been higher medical costs and simultaneous pressure to expand and increase Medicare coverage. As a result, Medicare has been expanded on an almost annual basis. The 1972 amendment extended benefits to disabled individuals regardless of age, and covered high costs of treating those with chronic kidney disease. Higher costs, however, have made the level of benefits provided by law inadequate.

It is time to take the next step: a total national health security program. It would seem reasonable to establish that as the goal and to phase into such a system as quickly as is feasible.

Being a recent supporter and an original sponsor of the Health Security Act proposal in the Senate, it has always seemed important to me that we establish the federal government's readiness to assure health care for all of our citizens. Sitting as Chairman of the Appropriations Subcommittee that handles health, I have been in a position to understand the health care crisis and its concern to the nation, and have come to feel that a commitment to action is absolutely imperative.

Recognizing that not all changes can be brought about at once, however, I introduced in 1971 a bill to immediately expand health care coverage for our children. But the time has passed for phasing into a national health program by selecting specific classes of health care recipients. Action for all our citizens is needed now. To the extent that a total protection system cannot be immediately created, it makes sense to at least establish such a system for our young and our old.

As mentioned earlier, the American public has begun to feel that the health care crisis cannot be solved by doctors alone, and to look to the federal government for assistance. As experience with the Medicare program has made abundantly clear, providing more federal money for health care is not enough. Simultaneous government attention must be paid to manpower and facility needs, to improved health delivery, and to a strong research effort in order to make the best use of federal dollars and to give Americans the best service for their money.

As one of the original sponsors of the proposed National Health Security Act, I also recognize that the workings of the legislative process may change some of its provisions. Thus, while total health coverage must remain our ultimate goal, it may be necessary to achieve that goal by gradual steps. One possibility is the creation of a public-private corporation along the lines of the Tennessee Valley Authority. In administering the insurance program, a corporation of this sort could combine the advantages of private incentives and public responsibility.

In seeking the best way to meet the goals of national health insurance, many questions must be faced. For example:

To what extent are health costs now covered by private health insurance and government health programs? In other words, what risks and expenses have to come out of the earnings and savings of consumers?

When public and private health insurance programs are available, are they adequate, or are there so many limitations that the protection is in reality insufficient or non-existent!

How is the burden of health care payment distributed? Are policies designed with the working man or corporate executive in mind? Will persons who will receive less expensive care pay the same price as those who will receive treatment through the best facilities? Will a person's ability to pay be reflected in his insurance permiums?

Are there enough facilities and sufficient manpower

to provide the care? Will there be sufficient doctors and nurses and other practitioners in the right places to meet the needs of the consumers?

Can we build a program of national health insurance that will create incentives for better care and increase the quality of care now given to consumers?

In conjunction with some initial universal health insurance program, Medicare could be expanded to include comprehensive coverage for children. This approach would maximize preventive care. and should be accompanied by protection for all individuals between ages 18 and 65 with coverage for medical catastrophies, and a set timetable to bring about universal comprehensive coverage.

Nearly all care for children is preventive, in that it either prevents a disease entirely, or prevents childhood illnesses and injuries from developing into more serious, lifelong disabilities. This was the essential thrust of the working paper legislation that I sponsored in 1971. It is crucial to recognize that pressing problems, especially major childhood illnesses, will continue to maim many children simply because their parents cannot afford proper medical treatment, leaving thousands of families destitute, with nothing but unpaid medical bills to show for years of savings.

Each year thousands of infants are born deformed, or die within the first year of life simply because they are born to low-income mothers who cannot afford proper maternal care for themselves or sufficient health care for their babies. The dimensions of this problem are shocking. For example, birth defects alone currently affect two and one-half million Americans under the age of twenty. The care of a child with a major defect, illness or injury generally entails prolonged hospitalization, care by a wide array of highly trained professionals, and expensive equipment. Medical bills rapidly mount into thousands of dollars, surpassing the coverage offered by even the best private insurance plans, and far outstripping all but the richest family's ability to pay.

An equally tragic picture is the plight of infants who are born every day into low-income families. Because women from these families so often cannot afford proper maternal care during their pregnancies, or adequate obstetrical care at the time of delivery, their babies far too often are born unhealthy as well as poor. The same poverty which denied their mother adequate maternal and obstetrical care continues to rob these infants of the health care which is so crucial in the first year of life. Scientific studies have shown that premature infants are especially apt to be born with major health problems, to be malnourished, and to die within their first year of life. While the national infant mortality rate is unacceptably high, approximately 20 deaths for every 1,000 births, the rate for babies of low-income parents is often more than twice as high. As a nation founded upon the dignity of human life, we should not tolerate this situation, where infants are maimed for life or often die for no other reason than that they and their mothers cannot obtain proper medical care.

A look at my own State of Washington helps to present the dimensions of the problem. Last year, approximately 4,000 Washington youngsters were being treated under the Crippled Children's Program, although the estimates by the State Director indicate that at least 16,000 children are in need of such treatment. This means that only about one-fourth of the children in Washington State who need treatment are receiving proper care. I am sure that the situation is no more encouraging in other states.

Certain principles ought to be established in judging the kind of national health insurance program that consumers in this country deserve. Such a set of principles should include the following:

First, there should be an opportunity for various groups in society to play a role in determining health policy and financing. Health care is too important to remain the sole province of any professional group, no matter how well-trained or well-intentioned. Therefore, ways ought to be found for employers and unions and general consumers to help determine the amount of money to be spent, efficiency of care, and priorities to be met first.

179

Because the government is now such a big purchaser of health services, it should be asking questions about what we are getting for our money. The same questions should be asked by consumers, because medical bills and taxes are increasing too rapidly.

Another important principle should be to ensure that the national health insurance program rewards physicians and practitioners and other organizations that are more productive, that use personnel in more innovative ways, and take advantage of new efficiencies and economies.

Another important principle to advance is the encouragement of preventive care. A system that puts money in a hospital's coffers or in a doctor's pockets only when someone gets sick does not encourage keeping people well. Such a system should include programs for health education, family planning, nutrition, and environmental concerns. It is clear that the most economical and humane method of dealing with illness is to prevent it.

Finally, it would make sense to establish the principle of accessibility to comprehensive and balanced care regardless of how rich a person is. The criterion should be whether or not the person requires medical care, and not whether he or she has enough money to afford it.

With these goals in mind, and in combination with a simultaneous and concerted effort in all other areas of the health care system, we should be able to establish within the immediate future a program to assure health security to all Americans at a reasonable cost.

12.　　　　　　　　　　　Environmental Health

The disease of lead-based paint poisoning is preventable. In its more severe forms, it can cause permanent brain damage and death. Treatment instituted at a severe or late stage of the disease is not effective in reversing such permanent brain damage.

So indicated Dr. J. Julian Chisolm, Associate Professor of Pediatrics at John Hopkins University in Baltimore. Dr. Chisolm has devoted most of his professional career to the study of lead exposure and lead poisoning in children, and has been an active member of several committees and panel considering various aspects of the problem.

Dr. Chisolm appeared before the Senate Committee on Labor and Public Welfare in March 1972, accompanied by two women whose children he had treated. One was Mrs. Emma Haskins:

I had a child and he was very active as an infant. The first thing I noticed was that he stopped talking. He was three and one-half years old when he stopped talking. We did not know exactly what was wrong with him when he first stopped.

I had taken him to a private doctor and he didn't know for sure what was wrong with him. At that time, I wasn't in the city. When I moved back to Maryland, I took him to the hospital here. They treated him at Johns

Hopkins. The doctors at that time didn't know for sure what was wrong with him. They gave him some medicine to calm him down because he was over-active, but this did not help. Two years leter, when he was six years old, he went into convulsions. That is when they discovered that he had lead paint poisoning.

The child is now ten years old, and he functions at a level between two years and three years old, but he is still not talking. He does not go to school; he has been in a state hospital for the retarded for over two years. Recently, I have been trying to get him home and to be able to go to a school for the handicapped riding a bus, coming back and forth home.

Mrs. Louise Burton related the story of her daughter, Valerie, to the Committee:

My daughter started losing weight. She started complaining, and I took her to the hospital and they couldn't do anything. In her final illness, she started to vomit and went into convulsions. Four days later, she went into a coma. She went into the hospital August 10 and she died August 29, and the doctor said that if she lived, she would have been blind. They worked on her all day, and they had to give her a brain operation. They told me that she was deaf and would never be able to talk anymore. I have another little girl five years old now. She still has lead in her. She goes and gets a blood check every three months. They say the paint usually doesn't peel, but it does. The paint is peeling off the walls now, and I live in the project.

Senator Harold Hughes of Iowa, a member of the Committee, questioned the witness further:

Senator Hughes: Do you live in a government project?
Mrs. Burton: Yes, and it contains lead because I carried it to the hospital and the doctor tested it.
Senator Hughes: Doctor, it seems in the instance of these two cases, the local physicians had

182

	difficulty diagnosing what was wrong. I do not know whether that was a result of further deterioration or what. To what extent are physicians alerted to look for the symptoms?
Dr. Chisolm:	I think this is quite variable. One of the big problems is that most of the hospitals in high-risk lead poisoning areas are staffed largely by young doctors just starting into medicine who have a lot of things to learn about besides lead poisoning.

The second thing is that lead poisoning does not show up in the usual source of laboratory tests. If you go to a hospital and have the usual chest x-ray or the usual blood count or urine specimen test, lead poisoning may not show up in these examinations. I think this is where the real diagnostic problem lies. You have to do special sorts of tests.

Senator Hughes: What are the symptoms of lead-based paint poisoning?

Dr. Chisolm: The early symptoms are a change in behavior. The child becomes irritable and fussy. He may vomit from time to time, and these are the sorts of things that are often passed off as a cold, as these mothers have mentioned.

They are passed off as being inconsequential and then you have, as both of these mothers represent, very chronic cases. For example, Mrs. Haskins' child stopped talking, and this was called a behavior disorder.

It has been proposed that homes be deleaded to protect the present generation of children. But what about the paint being put on the walls today? If we don't move now to make sure that it is non-leaded, then the present situation will be repeated thirty years from now. It is not enough to put a warning on a can of leaded paint, or to permit some household uses of leaded paint, for two reasons. First, householders might purchase leaded paint for one purpose and then finish using the contents of a can for painting a child's room or some other location accessible to the child. Second, children have been known to eat flaking chips of paint from the exterior of their homes.

A report of the New Haven Health Department estimates that one-third of the children poisoned by paint in New Haven, Connecticut ingested paint from exterior surfaces. Such situations led me to propose that the Lead-Based Paint Poisoning Amendment of 1972 contain standards that would set the maximum lead content of paint at 0.06 percent. I also remarked on the necessity for authorizing money for researching the problem. There is a need for better data on the extent of lead paint poisoning. We must develop better methods of screening children and homes for lead, and develop new ways of deleading.

Public health problem such as lead in the environment must be included in our comprehensive program to ensure adequate protection to the nation's children. We must prevent the tragedies that Mrs. Burton and Mrs. Haskins have so vividly described.

Once again, despite the fact that the Lead-Based Paint Poisoning Prevention Act authorized $30 million for budget years 1971 and 1972, the Nixon Administration requested no money for budget year 1971, and only after great pressure did they ask for a budget request of $2 million for budget year 1972. This amount, of course, is woefully inadequate to meet the need.

The Department of Health, Education and Welfare has estimated the tragic toll which lead paint poisoning exacts from the two and one-half million children who are now at risk in the lead belts of our cities: 600,000 can be expected to have elevated blood-lead levels. 50,000-100,000 will require medical treatment; 6,000 will become severely retarded, and

150 will require lifetime care. In addition, 200 will die each year from this completely avoidable disease.

The number of affected children may even be significantly larger than we had thought. There is surprising news that lead paint poisoning exists outside the inner city slums of our oldest cities. Cases have also been found in small towns, west coast cities, and other unsuspected areas. The resulting additionally exposed population could conceivably be as large as 600,000 youngsters.

We in the Congress must sound the call for action so that we can estimate how and how much money needs to be spent. For example, screening each child at risk in the lead belts of our country would cost significantly less than a massive program to remove the hazard. There are approximately thirty million dwelling units in the United States with lead paint on the walls, of which approximately seven million are deteriorating or dilapidated.

The problem of forcing deleading of houses is more appropriately dealt with at a local level through new or existing housing or building codes. However, since the problem is so acute and afflicted children are crying out for action, and the progress on the local level has not been all that could be expected, it may well be that the federal government must become more active in providing program grants to these localities.

As the example of lead paint poisoning indicates, health protection is more complicated now than ever before. Environmental hazards must be considered and eliminated wherever possible. Most protection areas have been a local responsibility, as for instance in fire provention, but because the problems have a significant deterimental effect nationally, wider attention needs to be focused on the problem. This concern led me to author a bill in 1973 that would create a federal program for fire prevention and control (FIREPAC).

The goal of this program is to assist state and local governments in reducing the incidence of death, personal injury and property damage from fire, and to increase the effectiveness and coordination of fire prevention and control agencies at all levels of government.

The 90th Congress established a National Commission on Fire Prevention and Control, which made an exhaustive and comprehensive examination of the nation's fire problems. This Commission made detailed studies of the extent of this problem in terms of human suffering and loss of life and property, and made several thoughtful recommendations, concluding that, while fire prevention and control is and should remain a state and local responsibility:

the federal government must ... help ... if any significant reduction in fire losses is to be achieved.

The Commission found that the United States today has the highest per capita rate of deaths from property loss from fire of all the major industrialized nations in the world. In fact, the United States death rate was 57.1 deaths per million, versus the 29.7 deaths per million for the next worse record held by our industrialized neighbor to the north, Canada.

I was particularly struck by one other major conclusion:

The striking aspect of the nation's fire problem is the indifference with which Americans confront the subject.

We as a nation should not be indifferent. Destructive fire takes a huge toll in lives, injuries, and property losses. Each year, 12,000 American lives are lost and $11 billion worth of our precious resources are wasted. Annual costs due to fire rank between crime and product safety in magnitude. Each year, 300,000 individuals are injured and 60,000 will spend anywhere from six weeks to two years recuperating. The real tragedy is that there are many measures — often very simple precautions — that can reduce these losses significantly.

My Fire Prevention and Control bill would be a first step toward combating this national neglect of the social and economic costs of fire. It should be made clear that, although a federal presence is needed in the fire prevention area, it should not "run the show". In fact, first prevention and control should remain primarily a local responsibility. Local governments have always shouldered this responsibility, they appreciate special local conditions and needs better than could an arm of the federal government. Therefore, the proposed program is to supplement rather than supplant any local effort. There are many aspects of the nation's fire problem that have not received enough attention — often due to a lack of resources. While genuine economic problems often stand in the way of deeper investment in fire protection, lack of understanding helps to account for the low priority given to fire protection.

The people to whom we turn when fire strikes — the volunteer and paid firefighter — have themselves been sorely neglected by the nation. Theirs is the most hazardous profession of all, with an injury rate of 39.6 per 100 men. Their training is often limited, their protective gear grossly inadequate, and their firefighting equipment archaic. It is to problems such as these that the Fire Protection and Control Act is addressed.

Classifying fire as an environmental health problem suggests several programs that could be instituted to improve the situation. These include the establishment of a research and development program, a fire data gathering system, fire prevention education, and the opportunity to establish master plans for fire prevention and control.

There is no reason that firefighters should not receive the same quality of training and teaching in advanced techniques and skills that the FBI Academy has provided for so many years to the nation's law enforcement officials. A Fire Prevention and Control Academy, if properly constituted, could serve not only as a national center for the education and training of firefighters, but also as a catalyst for modernization of fire prevention and control techniques. Although many state and local jurisdictions have established fire training centers, the quality of these centers varies throughout the nation, and a FIREPAC academy could play an important role in upgrading the curriculum of local programs.

The Commerce Committee hearings revealed that a major factor contributing to the high injury rate of firefighters is the antiquated personal protection equipment which they are forced to use. It should be possible through a research program to design equipment to alleviate many of these deficiencies.

The most important part of fire prevention is its human aspect. Fire kills, and for those who survive fire injuries, there is often a long, painful, and difficult recovery. About one-half of the victims of fire are children. The average hospital stay for a burn victim is over three times that of a medical or surgical patient. Their scars, psychological as well as physical, often last a lifetime.

At present, fewer than 100 of the 7,000 general hospitals in the United States provide specialized burn care. Together, these hospitals treat only 8 percent of those afflicted with serious burn injuries. In budget year 1972, the National Institutes of Health spent only $1.25 million on research connected with burns and their treatment. The Social Rehabilitation Service, an arm of HEW, spent an additional $380,000 on special studies on the rehabilitation of burn patients. This is grossly inadequate. The Fire Prevention and Control Act would authorize and direct NIH to undertake an expanded program of research on burns, treatment of burn injuries, and rehabilitation of victims of fires.

In studying the National Commission on Fire Prevention and Control Report, it becomes evident that the programs described in this proposed legislation could achieve a reduction of 5 percent a year in deaths, injuries, and property losses. This would mean that during the first ten years, 119,000 Americans would be spared the trauma of serious burn injury, and 8,300 lives would be saved. This appears to be a proper and prudent investment in an important environmental health problem.

Food Safety

Another area of public health that has received insufficient attention is the need to protect the public against unsafe foods as well as to ensure them of adequate nutrition.

In June 1973, I introduced a bill to strengthen the Food

and Drug Administration powers protecting the public against the serious problem of adulterated foods.

The Center for Disease Control (CDC) reports a total of 7,628 isolations of salmonella for the third quarter of 1972 — a weekly average of 587. Salmonella is only one form of food-borne disease, of which over 45,000 cases were isolated in 1972. The enormity of this problem is accentuated by the fact that the reported incidence undoubtedly understates the number of actual cases of food poisoning.

The purpose of my bill is to guide the Food and Drug Administration (FDA) in establishing levels of surveillance, and to provide a mechanism through which concerned members of the public and the scientific community can share in making new regulations and challenge them if they are inadequate. This will give the Food and Drug Administration access to the knowledge and expertise of outside scientists, and further secure the public's right to use unadulterated food.

The General Accounting Office (GAO) issued a report in 1972 on unsanitary conditions in the food manufacturing industry, pointing out that the FDA lacks authority to require registration of food plants. The report noted that the FDA orders inspections based on its inventory of food establishments, but this inventory is largely inaccurate. Without the authority to obtain a complete inventory, FDA cannot inspect all establishments, nor can it trace all potential sources of a problem once it has been identified with a particular food or processing procedure.

Food adulteration is most effectively controlled at the processing plant by quality-conscious manufacturers. This self-regulatory approach has been successful, but the frequent discovery of large batches of adulterated food indicates that the food industry and the public would well benefit from legislation giving the federal government greater authority to supervise and inspect the manufacture of this nation's food.

In perspective, food adulteration should be viewed as part of the need for a more general concern for food as a public health problem. Attention at the federal level should be paid to the relationship between nutrition, diet, and tooth decay, constipation, diabetes, obesity, intestinal cancer, hypertension, and heart disease.

Recent scientific studies indicate that many widely used food additives may not be as safe as has been asserted. Some of this new scientific evidence has resulted from new techniques used for detecting poisonous effects of chemicals on men and animals. The July 25, 1973 edition of the *Medical Tribune* described work done by Dr. Ben Feingold and a team of investigators in San Francisco, reporting that behavioral disturbances in children are probably the most important and dramatic of all the adverse reactions attributable to food additives. The resulting clinical problem is called "hyperkinesia", or over-activity which interferes with the child's attention span and is reflected in disruptive behavior both at home and at school. Dr. Feingold, of the Kaiser Foundation Hospital in San Francisco, told the Section on Allergy at the AMA Convention that these children suffer from an impaired ability to concentrate, and this leads to learning difficulties despite normal or high IQs. These children are:

baffling to psychiatrists, pediatric neurologists, psychiatrists, psychologists, and educators in the field of hyperkinesia and learning difficulty.

Dr. Feingold reported:

We have successfully treated some of these children with salicylate-free diet which eliminates 80 percent of the food additives including the artificial flavors and colors.

Children who have been put on this diet eliminating most of the food additives have become well-adjusted, both at home and at school.

Dr. Feingold described an average child's breakfast as follows:

a cereal loaded with non-essential flavors and colors added to entice a child, a beverage, either chocolates or other drinks, most of which are rich with many artificial colors, pancakes made from a mix, frozen waffles dyed with tartrazine, or frozen French toast. Then the conscientious and concerned mother gives the child vitamins, usually chewable, which are also loaded with additives. At school, the same ritual is continued at lunch. The child receives hot dogs, luncheon meats, ice cream and various beverages. Is it any wonder that our children are jumping and failing to learn?

One must be quick to point out that much more scientific evidence and corroboration are needed before food additives can be so directly linked to childhood behavioral disturbances. On the other hand, we should not sit around waiting for definitive proof that food additives really are harmful. The most prudent course would be to give the Food and Drug Administration sufficient muscle to look into such matters.

An even more recent study undertaken at Georgetown University is collaboration with the National Institutes of Health shows that some chemical compounds used to preserve beverages and canned and frozen foods can be harmful to human cells.

Reported in August 1973 in the Proceedings of the National Academy of Science, the study showed that several food additives commonly used to prevent food spoilage caused by bacteria and other disease-producing microbes act just as strongly against human and animal cells as they do against bacteria. In tissue culture studies, the additives were shown to inhibit cell growth, to alter the shape of certain cells, and in some cases, to destroy them. "Further study is necessary," Dr. T. Sreevalsan, Associate Professor at Georgetown University, was quick to point out. "But present evidence would urge caution in eating large quantities of food containing such additives."

Again, research has not come to a definitive conclusion, but if we are to protect the public from harmful foods on the market, health areas of this sort must be explored more closely than in the past.

The questions of food adulteration and the need for better surveillance and inspection of food raises the major

191

health problem of nutrition. Senator Ernest F. Hollings of South Carolina, an able colleague on our Senate Commerce Committee and a very active member of the Select Committee on Nutrition and Human Needs, has been in the forefront on this problem. In his fine book, *The Case Against Hunger,* Senator Hollings discusses how medical science has exposed the problem of nutritional deficiencies but has not solved it by any means. He has made us all aware that there is a strong relationship between nutrition and the human brain, and that citizens, because of a lack of nutrition, can be adversely affected for life.

One of the most important problems lies in nutritional deficiencies associated with pregnancy. It is during this period of major brain growth that a shortage of protein can greatly interfere with normal development, causing permanent brain damage or mental slowness, and leaving the child to enter the world with a lifelong handicap.

Dr. Charles Upton Lowe, Chairman of the Committee on Nutrition of the American Academy of Pediatrics, testified before a Senate committee that lack of nutrition can cause as much as a 20 percent loss in brain cell development. He then pointed out another distressing factor, premature births, in which as many as 50 percent of such infants grow to maturity with an intellectual competence significantly below normal. There is no doubt that severe malnutrition of young infants produces significant brain damage. Dr. Myron Winich of New York Hospital described the problem:

> First, this is a self-perpetuating problem, a vicious cycle which begins in infancy and condemns a person to a lifetime of perhaps marginal function, making it that much more difficult for him to extricate himself from the existing conditions; and it creates for his family an environment which will not protect his children from the same disease.

There have been several studies that reveal that poverty diets lack protein, and especially high quality protein. The question of diet and nutrition recalls vividly to mind the crisis in Seattle in 1972, when massive unemployment resulted from Boeing's cutback on jobs. The situation became so critical that thousands of engineers, scientists, and other employees were suddenly without work and reduced to bare subsistence levels. The community rallied admirably, but thousands of families were threatened by a need for food. After strenuous activity on the part of Senator Henry Jackson of Washington and myself, we were able to amend the existing Food Stamp program to supply surplus food to the families in need. This kind of situation leads me to feel even more strongly that we must do whatever we can to ensure that Americans have sufficient food, high in nutrition and free of harmful additives.

Another area requiring consumer protection is that of flammable fabrics.

In *The Dark Side of the Marketplace,* I gave the reasons that led me to author and introduce the Flammable Fabrics Act. Once a law is passed, making sure that it is implemented is every bit as important as enactment of the law itself. Therefore. I pay very strict attention to two aspects of the follow-through. The first is to make sure that the program gets enough money to carry out its mission. The second is to keep an eye on the program's results. Too often, agencies get swept up with reporting their activities, rather than reporting their results. This brings about too much bureaucracy and not enough results to the consumer.

A story in the June 6, 1973 *Seattle Times* caused me to be both angry and frustrated. It described Terri Patnode, age 5, of White Swan, Yakima County, who was brought to Children's Orthopedic Hospital the previous day with burns over about 75 percent of her body. Her flannel nightgown had ignited on contact with a gas stove flame at her home, and she had been treated at the Yakima Hospital and brought to Children's by ambulance in critical condition.

There were already laws on the books about flammable fabrics, but their implementation had been too slow to prevent Terri's accident. The *Yakima Republic* on June 9, 1973, had an editorial entitled, "What Price Safety?" This editorial put its finger on the problem, namely, "administrative and bureaucratic dilly-dallying for agonizing years — during which children were severely or fatally burned every day —".

It was precisely because of this bureaucratic delay that we insisted in Congress that this important protective law be taken out of the Department of Commerce and be placed in the new Consumer Product Safety Commission. The *Yakima Republic* editorial summed it all up as follows:

> Terri's case is only one of many, of course. But her suffering and that of her parents is just one more tragic demonstration of the price which consumers have to pay when bogged down administrators and stalling manufacturers play their crude and dangerous game.

The passage of a law for occupational health and safety further demonstrates the importance of implementation. In May 1971, the Nixon Administration issued a so-called "white paper" entitled, "Toward A Comprehensive Health Policy for the 1970s." Under the heading of prevention, this report indicated that prevention of deaths, illness and injury is a major part of the Administration's strategy. On-the-job accidents resulted in 14,500 deaths and more than two million disabling injuries during 1970. Gruesome statistics such as these led to the passage in that year of the Occupational Health and Safety Act. Under this law, the Secretary of Labor could implement existing safety standards and establish other federal standards for the promotion of occupational health and safety. The Act also authorized emergency action in the event of grave dangers from toxic agents or new hazards and established strict enforcement and inspection measures. It also set up a National Institute for Occupational Health and Safety within HEW to conduct research and experiments that would lead to new and improved standards.

In July 1973, Kenneth Peterson and George Taylor of the AFL-CIO appeared before our Senate Health, Education, and Welfare Appropriations Subcommittee. Mr. Peterson stated:

194

The AFL-CIO is appalled by the cuts of the Occupational Safety and Health Act (OSHA) affecting the progress of America.

Mr. Taylor indicated that organized labor was appearing before the Committee in a broad and urgent appeal to the Congress to save the Occupational Safety and Health Act of 1970 and to provide it with the guidance and resources necessary for carrying out its mandate to guarantee a safe and healthy workplace for every American working man and woman.

OSHA was designed to stop needless killing, maiming, and occupational diseases in the nation's workplaces. The magnitude of this problem cannot be overstated. A recently commissioned Department of Labor study indicated that accurate reporting would show an annual toll of 25,000 deaths and 20-25 million injuries to workers on the job. Furthermore, the Public Health Service estimates that, even with the present lack of precision in reporting occupational illnesses, we can expect at least 100,000 deaths and about 400,000 new cases of occupational disease each year. Mr. Peterson went on to state:

The budget proposal of the Nixon Administration for implementation of OSHA reflects mistaken policies which run counter to the intent of Congress when it passed the 1970 Act and can only result in the tragic delay of the preventive programs which this body placed into the statute.

On April 19, 1973, Dr. Marcus Key, Director of the National Institute for Occupational Safety and Health, stated at a meeting of the National Advisory Committee on Occupational Safety and Health:

NIOSH is not expanding; it is shrinking. It is getting the proverbial meat axe, in that a reduction in force is under way in our agency. Our present laboratory space isn't even adequate for any kind of research. It is substandard. We have been frozen on hiring for most of our

195

existence, and we are losing key staff right and left because we don't have the grade points to promote them. We can't compete with industry, we can't compete with other government agencies that have higher grade point averages. I don't think NIOSH is a viable organization at this time.

These are the words of the Nixon Administration Director of the program.

What has been true of the cancer program, where it is clear that the Administration is selling the public short, is also true of implementation of the Occupational Safety and Health Act. But this area is too important to be written off and dismissed. The public information required under the Act must be put forth, as well as the setting of standards required under this Act, and we should get on with the job of protecting the working men and women of this country. To do any less is a national disgrace. We must assure every worker that job-related injury and illness are not the penalties of working for a living.

The Senate Commerce Committee, and particularly the Subcommittee for Consumers, has been increasingly preoccupied with the pursuit of consumer health protection and safety. We have learned that, in order to make a significant impact on such major threats to health as lung cancer, emphysema, heart disease and automobile accidents, we must modify related social and environmental factors to protect against injury and illness, rather than allow the current state of medical care to continue. There is no doubt that our ability to change present patterns of cigarette smoking, air pollution, obesity and faulty road and automobile engineering holds great potential for the saving of lives and the prevention of pain and suffering. In the long run, emphasis on what are relatively inexpensive preventive measures can spare the incredible human costs which the nation currently incurs. Taking such measures now will also reduce the large losses in productivity that result when injured people are kept from working, and will prevent them from being a drain on our resources, rather than productive members of society.

Preventive health takes many forms. A single innovation such as an air-bag restraint system may well reduce deaths from automobile accidents by the thousands and the number of crippling injuries from automobiles by hundreds of thousands. Veils of secrecy are often the greatest problem in advancing causes that are in the public interest. Congress and the public must be kept fully informed and made welcome as participants in all of these areas of preventive health. To date, the voice of the citizen has never come close to receiving access to government equal with the voice of industry.

The federal government is in the consumer protection business to stay. Its efforts are already seen in the legislation creating a number of categorical programs, such as toy safety, flammable fabrics, refrigerator safety, poison prevention packaging, hazardous substances and electronic radiation. Congress has usually moved into these areas very slowly, only after very obvious and well-publicized hazards, and usually long after charred or mutilated bodies had begun to pile up high.

The creation of a Consumer Product Safety Commission has changed this significantly. It is hoped that this Commission will be independent of political and economic pressures, and that its focus will be on assuring the consumer and the public that the products they purchase will be safe and reliable. This Commission can enter and set standards in problem areas well before the damage is done, but to do an effective job, it needs much greater public support than in the past. I hope that this support will be forthcoming.

One of the important tasks of the 1970s and beyond will be to allow consumers a voice in setting standards in those areas that intimately affect them. This certainly includes all products that we purchase. We have not had sufficient balance between the voice of the consumer and the voice of industry with respect to protecting the health, safety and welfare of our citizens. We must build citizen awareness and allow for citizen advocates, both within and outside of the government, so that regulations and standards established in the public interest are not subverted.

An agency should not only have the power to set adequate safety standards, but also the power and the resources to make sure those standards are being met. The power to obtain access to important records and to inspect manufacturing premises when necessary is also necessary. We must not lose sight of the end product of the health care and delivery system, and that is the individual patient. Far too often, people get caught between the cracks, and never get the kind of care they need when they need it.

The areas of preventive health and environmental health protection are usually not dramatic. Consumers have not generally demanded protection, and thus it has been difficult to find a definite focus where demands can be met. But problems such as lead poisoning, fire protection, a safe workplace, and concern about food and nutrition are areas in which consumers need the government to establish standards. In the long run, basic measures taken in these areas can be as important as medical research and the practice of good medicine in improving the health of our citizens.

13.

"There is nothing so far removed from us as to be beyond our reach, or so hidden that we cannot discover it."   Rene Descartes 1637

Can we wipe out the major crippling diseases such as heart disease, cancer and stroke? If we can, we will have eliminated not only these dread diseases but the fear associated with them. I am convinced that we can make great headway against many of these killers.

Medical scientists appearing before Congress have indicated that we need not die by default from some debilitating disease. Dr. Lewis Thomas, President of Memorial Sloan-Kettering Cancer Center, appeared before our Senate Health Appropriations Subcommittee in February 1972:

I see no reason to suppose that heart condition is a natural part of the human condition, and I am convinced that cancer will eventually be entirely curable. I believe that we should be able to rid ourselves of the disabling diseases associated with aging, particularly stroke. There is one last problem which arises when medical scientists talk the way I am talking. What will we all die of? Without our major diseases, will we just go on and on with disastrous effects on the population problem? This

199

seems to be a non-problem. We will continue to age, wear out, and die; we will probably die according to the genetic schedules which we have inherited, some earlier, some later. I am not sure that our total life span will be greatly increased; some of us will live longer, obviously, but probably not the majority. What is certain is that the quality of life will be measurably improved, and old age will be changed from the floundering disaster which it now represents for so many people into something more like a natural human condition. It is worth the effort, it seems to me. Indeed, I am not sure that we can afford, for the long run, any other course.

For those of us who have been strong supporters of medical research, these words promise the fulfillment of our dreams. Major health breakthroughs that have occurred in the relatively short time that the National Institutes of Health have been in existence give me hope that our dreams will become reality — that all of the remaining disabling diseases will be cured. It would certainly be a much different and more pleasant world, especially for our elderly citizens, to know that they can remain productive and happy and healthy throughout their lifetimes. It could certainly change the perspective of growing old for all of us.

The elimination of dreaded diseases will not only improve the quality of our lives, it will also save us money. When a final breakthrough comes in a cure for a disease, it is generally in the form of a drug or vaccine that is relatively inexpensive and easy to deliver. It is certainly a good deal less expensive to prevent or cure an illness than it is to manage or contain it.

Today, however, preventive care alone cannot eliminate many debilitating diseases. As emphasized time and time again in this book, the only way for us to ever cure such diseases as heart attack, stroke, and cancer will be through research breakthroughs that must have their origin in the laboratory. If we are going to make long-term, permanent progress in health care in the 1970s and beyond, our highest priority must be to provide significant resources for medical research.

In spite of the number of major diseases that cannot be greatly helped by prevention and screening, there are of course a number of important areas of prevention that can facilitate good health. This book points out several of these areas and shows why the federal government must be concerned about these issues and problems. Many of these issues concern personal health services in which government must make certain that resources, manpower and technology are used to provide consumers with the latest information and treatment available. As was pointed out earlier in the book, there are several communicable diseases, including polio, diphtheria, whooping cough and other contagious diseases that can now be prevented. The government must encourage prevention and screening of personal health services for citizens particularly through the development of health maintenance organizations or any other efficient, economic, and high quality delivery system.

In addition to the areas of preventive medicine over which an individual has some control, there are many areas beyond his direct control which must be dealt with by society as a whole. As more and more of the detrimental aspects of the environment become known, it becomes more important for government to take a role in establishing standards to deal with them. Government must see to it that the water our citizens drink is safe, that the air they breathe is clean, that their workplaces are not hazardous to their health, and that consumer products including such items as automobiles, toys, fabrics and other products are as safe as our technology can reasonably make them.

The 1970s and beyond will see a growing dependence upon the government to secure the safety of all these items for the public. There is no doubt that the Consumer Product Safety Commission will become one of the most important protective agencies in this country. It will take the next few years for the Commission to assimilate all of the varied tasks that have been assigned to it by Congress. Those of us instrumental in its establishment will watch it carefully to make sure it carries out its tasks faithfully in the public interest.

Government has always had a responsibility for protecting the health, safety, and welfare of its citizens, but the federal government must do yet more to establish baseline standards for protecting the public. The advances made by the Commerce Committee in such areas as consumer product safety, fire prevention and no-fault automobile insurance are prototypes of creative ways that the federal government can protect consumers. The Fire Prevention and Control Program, for example, is to assist state and local governments in reducing the incidence of death, personal injury and property damage from fire, as well as to increase the effectiveness and coordination of fire prevention and control agencies at all levels of government. The program will keep fire prevention and control where it belongs, namely, at the state and local level, but allow the federal government to supplement, without supplanting state and local efforts. As an example, the proposed Fire Prevention and Control Academy will serve as a national center for the education and training of fire fighters, and also promote the modernization of fire prevention and control techniques.

As this nation moves further and further to control and, in some cases, cure major diseases, an equal effort must be made to prevent environmental and accidental hazards. It makes no sense to keep people from succumbing to disease only to have them be needlessly exposed to environmental dangers that could be eliminated by present or future technology.

In the rest of this decade and beyond, the federal government must assume greater responsibility for protecting the consumer and his health needs. When only seven of the 127 water systems in the State of Washington can pass bacteriological standards for safe drinking water, then it is time for positive action. We need a system of national drinking water standards to protect the public health. When more sophisticated testing finds viruses and toxic organic compounds in drinking water even after it has been "completely treated," then it is time to establish standards that will upgrade the quality of water treatment.

I agree with Ralph Nader in ranking water contamination as one of the top five consumer issues in the United States today. I believe that a United States citizen should expect that the water he drinks and the air he breathes will do him no harm. Congress over the next several years must work diligently to guarantee this right to our citizens.

Consumers must also be protected from poor quality products, whether they be unsafe toys or unsafe medical devices or unsafe health practitioners or facilities. The Professional Standards Review Organizations (PSRO) recently legislated by Congress is a start in this direction.

Unnecessary pain and suffering and even risk of death through unnecessary operations must be stopped. Organized medicine, through the PSRO concept, has asked to be given the opportunity to police the quality and cost of medical care. But, as has been indicated often in this book, the establishment of standards does not guarantee improvements in quality. Incentives must be built in and bureaucratic red tape must be eliminated.

The most important health issue this country must face over the next several years is why any man, woman, or child in this country should go without lifesaving health care, especially if the limiting factor is inability of that person to pay for such care. Members of Congress receive letters from constituents asking sometimes confusedly, and other times with blunt fury, why, if our health research is second to none and if we have many of the world's most sophisticated clinics and hospitals, the average taxpayer cannot receive the best care at a reasonable cost?

Even with higher and higher costs, medical care has become increasingly difficult to obtain, and larger areas of the population are seriously underserved. Despite larger expenditures by the consumer out of his own pocket, comprehensive health care has not been made available and health insurance coverage still has far too many loopholes.

A national health insurance plan must be established on the premise that quality health care be assured to all our citizens. That the federal government will be spending close to $80 billion for health by 1980 if we continue with the current health system, in comparison to $33 billion being spent in 1974, should be a powerful incentive to founding a more efficient health care delivery system. It is equally essential that the federal government fulfill its responsibilities in research, health manpower training, and the maintenance of adequate facilities. A well-conceived health insurance plan that enables the consumer to purchase care will not discover a cure for heart disease, train more doctors, build additional mental health centers, or better organize our health resources. National health insurance will offer only an empty promise of health care unless we meet these responsibilities as well.

In order for national health insurance to keep its promise, consumers must be assured of a sufficient number of physicians and other health practitioners. The current health manpower shortage is quite serious, and steps must be taken immediately to make sure there will be enough doctors a decade from now. The United States is importing over 5,000 foreign-trained doctors each year, and one-third of all doctors in residency training received their basic medical education in foreign schools. This dependence on other countries leads to serious questions about the quality of health care, now and in the future.

For millions of Americans living in small rural towns and urban areas, the physician problem is even more basic. Ways must be found to encourage physicians and other health personnel to leave the large metropolitan areas where they receive their training, and go to the small towns where people are, quite literally, dying because they cannot get to a doctor soon enough after a heart attack, or after a tractor turns over and crushes the driver. The National Health Service Corps could be one answer to this pressing manpower problem. The Corps must, however, receive administrative support and incentives to make it work. Otherwise, health problems that are routine and trivial in richer communities will continue to be serious or fatal for those who do not have adequate access to doctors.

In order to provide the citizens of this country with the first-rate health care system they deserve, all of the different pieces — research, manpower training facilities, environmental protection, consumer safety — must be linked in a strong chain that will get the researcher's findings to the sick or injured American's bedside, whether he is in Beverly Hills or Stevenson, Washington. This care and protection must be brought to each and every American citizen, regardless of how much money he has. After all, in the final analysis, that is all that counts.

Bibliography

Much of the source material for this book comes from personal knowledge, communications, letters, and interviews. However, the reader who would like to explore the subject further may consult a number of excellent sources. The authors found the following articles, books, and publications especially valuable in preparing this book.

Anlyan, William G. "Will Partisan Politics Determine the Nature and Quality of Health Care?" *New England Journal of Medicine,* vol.286, June 1, 1972:1184-1186.

Chapman, Carleton B. and John M. Talmadge. "Historical and Political Background of Federal Health Care Legislation." *Law and Contemporary Problems.* vol.35, spring 1970:334-347.

Committee for Economic Development. *Building a National Health Care System.* New York, 1973.

Cray, Ed. *In Failing Health; the Medical Crisis and the A.M.A.* Indianapolis, Bobbs-Merill Co., 1970.

Edwards, Marvin Henry. *Hazardous to your Health.* New Rochelle, N.Y., Arlington House, 1972.

Ehrenreich, Barbara and John. *The American Health Empire: Power, Profits and Politics.* New York, Vintage Books, 1971.

Falk, I.S. "National Health Insurance: a Review of Policies and Proposals." *Law and Contemporary Problems,* vol.35, autumn 1970.

Fried, Edward R., Alice M. Rivlin, Charles L. Schultze,

Nancy H. Teeters. *Setting National Priorities, The 1974 Budget,* Washington, D.C., the Brookings Institution, 1973.

Garfield, Sidney R. "The Delivery of Medical Care." *Scientific American,* vol.22, April 1970:15.

Gerber, Alex. *The Gerber Report.* New York, McKay, 1971.

Glazer, Nathan. "Paradoxes of Health Care." *Public Interest,* no.22, winter 1971:62-77.

Gorman, Mike. "Impact of National Health Insurance on Delivery of Health Care." *American Journal of Public Health,* vol.61, May 1971:962-971.

Inglehart, John K. "Executive–Congressional Coalition Seeks Tighter Regulation for Medical Services Industry." *National Journal,* November 1973:1684-1692.

Kennedy, Edward M. "Health Care in the Seventies." *Journal of Medical Education,* vol. 47, Jan. 1972:15-22.

_____. *In Critical Condition.* New York, Simon and Shuster, 1972.

Magnuson, Warren G., and Jean Carper. *The Dark Side of the Marketplace: The Plight of the American Consumer.* Englewood Cliffs, N.J., Prentice Hall, 1968.

_____. "Congressional Responsibility for Preventive Health Care." *Preventive Medicine,* vol.3, August 1972.

Milbank Memorial Fund Quarterly. Health and Society. vol.51, nos. 2&3, spring, summer 1973.

National Commission on Product Safety. Final Report Presented to the President and Congress. 1970.

Olson, Stanley W. "Health Insurance of the Nation." *New England Journal of Medicine,* vol.284, March 11 1971:525-535.

Pettengill, Daniel W. "Writing the Prescription for Health Care." *Harvard Business Review,* vol.49, Nov-Dec 1971:37-43.

Pollack, Jerome. "Raising the Curtain and the Sights of National Health Insurance." *Hospital Management.* vol.110, August 1970:32.

Randal, Judith, and others. "The High Cost of Health" (series). *Washington Evening Star,* Jan-Mar 1970.

Ribicoff, Sen. Abraham with Paul Danaceau. "The American Medical Machine." New York, *Saturday Review Press,* 1972.

Rogers, David E. "The Unity of Health: Reasonable Quest or Impossible Dream?" *Journal of Medical Education,* vol.46, Dec. 1971:1047.

Schorr, Daniel. *Don't Get Sick in America.* Nashville and London, Aurora, 1970.

Schwartz, Harry. *The Case for American Medicine.* New York, McKay, 1972.

Somers, Ann R. *Health Care in Transition.* Chicago Hospital Research and Educational Trust. 1971.

Strickland, Stephen P. *Politics, Science, and Dread Disease.* Cambridge, Harvard University Press, 1972.

U.S. Congress. House. Committee on Ways and Means. *Basic Facts on the Health Industry.* 92nd Congress, 1st Sess.

U.S. Congress. Senate. Committee on Appropriations. H.R.8877. *Hearings on the Department of Health, Education, and Welfare Appropriations for Fiscal Year 1974* May, June 1973.

U.S. Congress. Senate. Committee on Commerce. S.1478. *Federal Hazardous Substances Act. Hearings before the Commerce Committee.* 92nd Congress, 2nd Sess. March 1972.

U.S. Congress. Senate. Committee on Commerce. S.426 and S.888. *Toxic Substances Control Act of 1973. Hearings before the Commerce Committee.* 92nd Congress, 2nd Sess. March 1972.

U.S. Congress. Senate. Committee on Commerce. S.354. *National No-Fault Motor Vehicle Insurance Act.* 93rd Congress, 1st Sess. Parts 1&2, April 1973.

U.S. Congress. Senate. Committee on Commerce. S.433 and S.1735. *Hearings before the Subcommittee on Environment.* 93rd Congress, 1st Sess. May 1973.

U.S. Congress. Senate. Committee on Finance. *Hearings on National Health Insurance.* 92nd Cong., 1st Sess. April 26, 27,28,1971.

U.S. Congress. Senate. Committee on Government Operations. Subcommittee on Executive Reorganization. *Health Care in America. Hearings,* 90th Cong., 2nd Sess. Parts 1-2, April-July 1968.

U.S. Congress. Senate. Committee on Labor and Public Welfare. *Lead-Based Paint Poisoning. Hearings Before the Subcommittee on Health.* 91st Cong., 2nd Sess. Nov. 23 1970.

U.S. Congress. Senate. Committee on Labor and Public Welfare. S.4106. *National Health Service Corps. Hearings before the Subcommittee on Health.* 91st Cong., 2nd Sess. Aug. 28 1970.

U.S. Congress. Senate. Committee on Labor and Public Welfare. National Program for the Conquest of Cancer. *Report of the National Panel of on the Conquest of Cancer.* 92nd Congress, 1st Sess. April 14 1971.

U.S. Congress. Senate. Committee on Labor and Public Welfare. S. 3080. *The Lead Paint Poisoning Prevention Act. Hearings before the Subcommittee on Health.* 92nd Congress, 2nd Sess. March 1972.

U.S. Congress. Senate. Committee on Labor and Public Welfare. S.3858 and S.3867. *Health Manpower Shortages. Hearings before the Subcommittee on Health.* 92nd Cong., 2nd Sess. Aug. 1972.

Vayda, Eugene. "Stability of the Medical Group in a New Prepaid Medical Care Program." *Medical Care,* vol.8, March 1970:161.